*The Revolutionary Diet Approach to
Eliminating Upper Respiratory Problems—
Including Children's Middle Ear Infections*

No More
allergies,
asthma
or sinus
infections

by Dr. Lon Jones

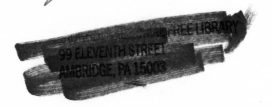

Book design by Bonnie Lambert.

ISBN 978-1-893910-88-1

Freedom Press, LLC
www.freedompressonline.com
Bulk Orders Available: (800) 959-9797
E-mail: info@freedompressonline.com

Advance Praise

"I hope every family doctor and pediatrician in America reads this book—for the sake of their patients!"
—Ronald L. Hoffman, MD, medical director of The Hoffman Center and host of the nationally syndicated radio program *Health Talk*

"*No More Allergies, Asthma, or Sinus Infections* offers a straight-forward, 'common sense' approach to anyone who suffers from the unbearable symptoms of respiratory tract challenges. This book is a 'must read' for the person in your life who suffers needlessly from these all too-common health challenges. It is a perfect patient education tool for every doctor in family practice today. It's as if Dr. Jones is in the room with you."
—Dr. David C. Kolbaba, natural healthcare practitioner and show host of *HealthQuest Radio* Chicago

"Xylitol is a very versatile compound that will help a lot of people. It has great potential as both a sweetener and for its use in dental health. Xylitol is also extremely effective, as we learn from Dr. Lon Jones, in its ability to cleanse the nasal cavity and sinuses and help us to deal with a myriad of respiratory health challenges. A highly recommended read for anyone dealing with these issues."
—Jordan S. Rubin, *The New York Times* best-selling author of *The Maker's Diet*

"I learned so much from Dr. Jones about the benefits of xylitol in a nose wash and how it reduces middle ear infections. As a dentist I was already aware of the anti-cavity benefits using xylitol and now parents and doctors can learn more from this very practical approach to better health."
—**Doyle Williams, DDS, Chief Dental Officer, DentaQuest**

"Don't let Dr. Lon Jones' self-proclaimed description, as being a rural Texas country doctor with a mission and simple message, lull you into not understanding that you're about to read a profound and light-years-ahead-of-its-time quality and quantity life-extending, self-help exposé. I consider Dr. Jones to be the modern day 'Father of Functional Nasology.' *No More Allergies, Asthma or Sinus Infections* should be required reading for all primary-care providers, including MDs, DOs DCs, NDs, all dental professionals as well as lay people. And in doing so, mankind is ultimately better served."
—**Robert C. Martin, DC, DACBN, author of** *Secret Nerve Cures* **and nationally syndicated host of** *The Dr. Bob Martin Show*

This book is dedicated to my mother, who died last year, and to my wife, Jerry Bozeman. My mother's daily admonishment as she sent me off to school was: "Keep your nose clean." When I got older I asked her whether the admonishment was metaphorical or real and she told me about a classmate of hers in grammar school who had a chronic runny nose and how it affected her relationships with classmates—it wasn't metaphorical. As I learned more about how the body works it always made sense to promote our cleaning defenses, so Mom's advice stayed with me; and the fact that I finally found a way to honor her request gave her some joy in her final years.

You will get to know more about Jerry in the book, but it was her experience in special education, and the connection that she observed between ear infections and learning problems that prompted her remark to me that changed everything: "If somebody really cared about children they would find a way to prevent ear infections." Having fathered several children of my own as well as being an adoptive, step, and foster father to more, that was a challenge I could not escape, especially when the recurrent ear infections that led to the discussion were in our granddaughter.

Contents

No More Upper Respiratory Problems

My name is Dr. Lon Jones. I guess you could call me a country doctor since I practiced in rural Texas.

I am also an osteopathic physician and more osteopaths turn out to be country doctors, or at least family physicians, than any other branch of medicine—and, oh yes, in case you're wondering we osteopaths are every bit the doctor that your M.D. is. We work a little differently but in the pantheon of medicine we are equally considered to be treating physicians. Back in the days when I was looking at medical schools I wasn't familiar with Osteopathic medicine, but I was not particularly attracted to the way medicine was taught and practiced in regular medical schools: the focus seemed to be more on the disease than the person who had it. Medical schools then took younger people so they could practice longer, but many were so young they were uncomfortable dealing with people so they went into the specialties, like radiology and pathology, where they didn't have to see patients at all, or other specialties that allowed them to focus on just a part of the patient. I wanted something better and when someone mentioned Osteopathic medicine and I read about it, it was more in line with what I wanted.

Osteopathic medicine tends to focus more on the person, while traditional medicine tends to focus more on the symptoms. A founding principle of Osteopathic medicine is that the body is able to heal itself if it has what it needs and everything is working well. For osteopathic physicians like me, a significant part of our institutional memory is the success we had in America treating people with the flu after World War I.

This flu epidemic killed millions of people around the world and the virus that caused it is closely related to the H1N1 strain that we are dealing with now, which is in part why there is so much concern about it today. But in 1919, those treated in the United States by Osteopathic physicians had a mortality rate that was twenty times less than those treated by regular physicians. Originally this was credited to their use of manipulation, the practice that seemed to characterize osteopathic physicians. But Dr. Harold Magoun, Jr., writing in the October 2004 issue of the *Journal of the American Osteopathic Association*, took another look. He pointed out that the standard treatment used by regular, allopathic physicians was aspirin to reverse the fever and cough suppressants to stop the cough. He remembered the osteopathic principle that the body can heal itself and he knew that a fever and a cough are both defenses that help us better cope with invading agents. Hobbling those defenses meant that those with the flu had less ability to cope with the virus. Osteopathic physicians used neither of these treatments; and saw a twenty fold increase in survival because the defenses of the individuals were better able to cope.

This book is not about osteopaths or osteopathic medicine, though that founding principle is in every page. It is about how we can help our defenses, particularly those in the nose, and how optimizing those defenses can virtually eliminate upper respiratory problems. This is our primary message.

There are also some other lessons that we will learn on the way. First of all, the way we see things in modern medicine is largely wrong headed. Before going to medical school I studied history, especially the history of ideas and science, which includes medicine. Western medicine has its roots in what is called humoral medicine. The Greeks and Romans thought that illnesses were caused by an imbalance of the humors and had treatments that were aimed at correcting the imbalance. Blood was one of the humors and when someone showed symptoms, like a fever, they were bled until the symptoms got better. It wasn't until the middle of the 19th Century that physicians got around to asking the right question about bloodletting: What does it do to life expectancy? They found that more people died after having been bled. If you ask most physicians about humoral medicine they will likely tell you that we don't practice that way anymore and that the studies on bloodletting are what killed it. But the culture of humoral medicine continues today; we have just changed the humors and made them more scientific. The focus remains on symptoms, our drugs are measured by what they do to the target 'humor' (blood pressure, glucose level, fever, . . . or whatever target is being addressed), not what it does to life expectancy.

Rather than focus on symptoms, we would be better off learning a lesson from the biologists. Biologists are asking why we have symptoms; and what they find is that many of them are defenses that are expressed in us because of natural selection and the fact that they have a significant survival benefit. We have a fever, as Dr. Magoun noted, because it helps us deal more effectively with infections—it's a defense that needs to honored and supported rather than just turned off; and biologists overwhelmingly agree. Most physicians know this too, but they haven't gotten around to agreeing.

The first lesson then is that we humans have defenses that help us better cope with the dangers in our environments and that many of them come with a survival benefit that western medicine has not even considered. Indeed western medicine has often continued in the humoral mode of balancing these symptoms with drugs that turn them off, without asking why they are there, and eliminating in the process their survival value. We hope this book will help change that and finally lay the humoral concept in its proper grave.

The second lesson paints with an even broader brush. While it is easy to see that some of our symptoms may be defenses, it is harder to see that we adapt. For close to three centuries now the focus of western science has been analytical. When something doesn't work right we take it apart, find the part that is broken, replace or repair it, and put it back together confident in our fix; and in the last three centuries most of what we have worked with has been mechanical where this method is appropriate. But increasingly, the systems we work with are not mechanical. The human body is not a simple mechanical device; it is not even a complicated mechanical device—and the difference is significant. Machines can be predicted; they can't adapt or create something new. Living agents can create novel solutions as they adapt to changes in their environments and are not reliably predictable. While there is much in the practice of medicine that is causally related we would be far better served if medical educators and researchers could be reoriented to seeing the human body as what is called a complex adaptive system rather than the mechanical model they erroneously, and exclusively, continue to use. The second lesson is common sense to everyone who thinks about: humans can adapt and they are not predictable. But scarce few of our institutions recognize and honor that fact, and medical education and research are in the middle of the pack, thinking that the human body can be analyzed, fixed by repairing broken parts, and is essentially seen as a mechanical device. We hope also that those reading this book will experience this reorientation. It is true and it is common sense.

I practiced medicine in the Texas panhandle where I saw a lot of patients with all sorts of problems; I must admit the whole gamut. But, I also have to say, the largest part of patients I saw had respiratory problems—from allergies and asthma to middle ear infections, colds and the flu. Even though the sinuses of adults and middle ears of children are not associated with breathing, they are adjacent to the upper airway, and their problems begin there, so they are classified as 'upper respiratory' as well. Indeed, studies tell us that my experience is not unique: upper respiratory problems such as these are the number one reason for visiting your doctor.

You would think that things might be different living out here in the middle of the largest of the lower states where we are free from urban pollution. But even here in rural Texas, we have enough pollution from agricultural use of fertilizers, aerial spraying, and dust storms—to say nothing of the dust from cotton gins—to have many of the same problems that we typically think of as occurring in highly urbanized and industrialized regions. In any event, upper respiratory problems are a major problem in the health of our people, just as they are in the rest of the nation. Because of the stories I am going to relate, I came to be known as the doctor you go to as your last resort when it comes to upper respiratory problems. Patients often came to me after they had exhausted just about every other avenue of treatment—after they or their children were prescribed drugs, multiple drugs, and often even after having surgery for their problem.

People came to me because I helped developed a nasal spray that strengthens and augments our normal nasal defenses, which helps patients stay healthy and does not involve the use of any drugs. It is a very simple and safe nasal spray, and has been proven effective in studies from throughout the world. It honors what my Mom told me every day: "Keep your nose clean!" She couldn't have been more right.

CHAPTER ONE

Heather

CASE 1

Heather is our granddaughter; her ear infections started all of this. She was breast fed until she was two years old and neither parent smoked, so she had little risk for ear infections. But when she was five months old, her parents placed her in day care so that Mom could return to teaching school, and within two months she had an ear infection. It was treated and resolved with antibiotics, but the infections returned; within five months she'd had four more. These were the circumstances that led to the development of our nasal spray and Heather's parents and day care workers really came through for her and us as we searched for a way to help.

Learning problems are associated with recurrent ear infections in this critical time of life. These problems occur even when ear infections are treated appropriately. And ventilation tubes placed in the eardrum to help the infections to drain do not help the learning process!

Heather's parents and day care workers understood the need for consistency. They cooperated in spraying her nose every time they changed her diaper. She had no further ear infections until about six months later when a new day care worker was hired who was not aware of the spraying routine. Reestablishing regular nasal washing resolved this problem without the need for antibiotics. She continues to use this spray on a regular basis and averaged less than one febrile episode a year throughout her four years in day care, far less than the six upper respiratory infections or URIs per year described as normal for children attending day care. Her only antibiotic use since has been when she had a sore throat and tested positive for strep.

CASE 2

Traci was nine and had asthma so bad that she was in the emergency room at least once a month near my offices in Hale Center. Traci was on five different medications for her asthma including systemic steroids that are known to block growth.

Asthma is such a difficult disease; seldom is a condition associated with such a profound and anxiety-producing threat as shutting down one's ability to breathe. And the drugs we use to treat it can be very toxic. Admittedly, they are not as toxic as they used to be before we could better select for relaxing the bronchial constriction without speeding up the heart rate as well. In those days, it seemed that almost as many people died from overdosing as from asthma; I even had a classmate in medical school that died from asthma drugs. Unfortunately, more and more asthma cases are being reported throughout the country, especially in urban areas, but also where there is a lot of agriculture.

Traci's mother wanted to know if the nasal spray my wife and I had recently developed for preventing Heather's ear infections would help her daughter. I told her it wouldn't hurt. The spray is actually very simple, something I'll tell you more about, including all of the scientific evidence, besides providing my own results from working with thousands of patients with respiratory challenges. But for now, just know that her mother put it in with all of her other medications and sprayed her nose with it four times a day. About a week later, Mom was washing Traci's hair when she began choking, coughing, and wound up vomiting.

Traci threw up a bunch of thick jelly-like tissue. Mom thought she was losing her brains. A week later though, Traci noticed that she didn't have any problem breathing. Two weeks later she was continuing to breathe really quite easily, so Mom and I decided to gradually stop her asthma medications. Still no problems. Six months later, Traci was playing basketball and doing gymnastics with no wheezing at all. But what does washing your nose have to do with asthma? Well, that's what I'm going to explore with you.

CASES 3-12

After Heather's story appeared in a local paper, I soon had many other similar children in my practice, and they came from all over the place. Their parents and grandparents living in our town read about Heather and told their children. I only saw these children a few times usually, so this is certainly not a study on resolving ear infections, but I was able to get follow-up information on how ten of them used the health care system. These children and their concerned parents are what I call my 'Ears and Fears' study. In the five months before I saw them, these ten children had been taken to the doctor and received antibiotics for ear complaints a total of 43 times. Over the average of eleven months that we watched these children, and their noses were washed just like Heather's, they went to the doctor for ear complaints and received antibiotics a total of seven times. That's a 92 percent reduction in doctor visits and antibiotic use. Actually it was even better than 92 percent because of the seven times they went to the doctor three were in one child and three occurred when the parents had run out of the spray.

Since all upper respiratory infections follow essentially the same pattern, with the bacteria first colonizing the nose and then spreading to other areas to trigger infections, results like these are the basis of our hope to eliminate upper respiratory problems. And it is not just children who benefit.

CASE 13

Beth was a teacher who loved teaching little children, but her extensive close contact with them also opened her up to getting lots of sinus infections. By the time she came to me, she had almost given up on the medical profession because the continuous use of antibiotics didn't seem to help. She even got to the point where she would wear a bandana tucked into her glasses to catch the sinus drainage when she bent over to help her students. After she started using the spray regularly her problem became much less, but she still had occasional episodes where she relied on her topical decongestants to help open her nose. For reasons that we will discuss later we don't think that is a good idea. Instead, we encouraged Beth to lie down for a few minutes on her back, put a few drops of our spray in each nostril, and wait a few minutes to allow the solution to get to the back of the nose. This seemed to do the trick and Beth has been free of problems ever since.

CASE 14

DC, 42, has had diabetes and asthma for about twenty years. She had been on multiple medications for her asthma, including steroids that made her diabetes harder to manage. She had been in the hospital for her asthma and related pulmonary infections an average of two times annually for the past ten years. She began using the spray regularly and in the ensuing year did not experience any asthma and did not require any asthma medication. After such a long time with asthma, DC's airway had remodeled to be narrower. Doctors dealing with chronic asthma argue that this remodeling is permanent. Peak flow is the amount of air the person can move as they breathe; it reflects the size of the airway. DC's peak flow remained at 150 to 200 L/min for about 6 months, which wasn't very good and reflected her remodeled airways, but it was 350 L/min after a year of regularly cleaning her nose.

CASE 15

Jim worked at the local meat packing plant in the warehouse. He drove a forklift and was in and out of the freezer all day long. The constant temperature change played havoc with his sinuses. He used a nasal decongestant for years, which enabled him to breathe easier, but seemed to make his nose worse. Within a week after beginning use of the spray he had "a new life."

These are just a few of thousands of people who have seen their upper respiratory problems—including middle ear infections, allergies, asthma and sinus infections—disappear when they began their nasal hygiene program. The spray doesn't do anything to the viruses or irritants that trigger our infections or allergies or asthma; it is not an offensive weapon like antibiotics. All it does is support our defensive team, a critical part of our game with the noxious and infectious elements in our environment.

As we should have learned earlier from our experience with the 1919 flu, strengthening your defensive team will help us to win the game that we are all playing with the infectious and noxious elements in our environments. To be sure, not everyone is cured so easily; many seem to get no benefit. We feel sure that getting to these people earlier, while their defenses are still intact, would enable them also to realize the benefits that thousands of others have experienced.

Most of us are cautioned about using superlatives like *no more..., or everyone*, or *all* to describe a condition that may not be that general—you know, "Never say, *never*." But I feel safe in saying that at some point everyone has had an upper respiratory infection.

Commonly called URIs, they are the most common complaint seen by primary care physicians. They are called *upper respiratory* infections because they begin there, in the back of the nose, where the respiratory tract begins, and where all of the pollutants and airborne infecting agents enter the body as we go through the cycle of breathing more than 10,000 times every day. Most URIs are caused by viruses, some by bacteria; many are caused by a combination because viral infections do seem to open the doors for more bacteria and vice versa; it's as if they intuitively and instinctively cooperate, knowing their biological interests are shared.

Colds and flu happen all year long, but in the temperate zones of the world they are much more concentrated in the fall and winter months—we call this cold and flu season. There is not a flu season in the tropics—and I will explain why. And while colds and flu affect everyone, they are more of a problem for the very young and the very old, where they can even kill.

As the examples above suggest, I also feel safe in saying that the vast majority, if not all, of these infections are unnecessary. In dealing with these infecting problems in the past, we have concentrated our efforts on stopping the agent. We have developed antibiotics that kill them, or immunizations that help our bodies kill them. We concentrate on the offensive aspects of this warfare and ignore the defenses we all have that help us to survive in the midst of our polluted and bacteria-laden world—indeed with the wonders of modern medicine we are more likely to hobble our defenses than help them.

We do this because that is how we think about our problems in medicine. Five hundred years ago, illness was thought to be caused by sinning or some other action that was wrong or against nature; illness came to us as punishment from the gods. But three hundred and fifty years ago a British physician named Thomas Sydenham turned this theory upside down. He lived during the last of the bubonic plagues and wrote about how different illnesses show similar patterns in different people. He thought ill-nesses came from something outside the body and his view came to be accepted over the years. It was given a tremendous boost when Louis Pasteur showed how anthrax was caused by a bacterium and proposed the germ theory of disease; germs from outside us caused disease. This view-point continues spreading as we find infections associated with ulcers, heart disease, even cervical and breast cancer.

Since then, we have concentrated our efforts on finding and eliminating these external agents. We have concentrated on the offensive, on finding ways to kill or incapacitate the opposition. James K. Galbraith coined the term 'conventional wisdom' to describe how a society comes to share a con-cept or a way of seeing an issue, and the view is always fostered by profit somewhere. So too the conventional wisdom in medicine, that focuses on the offensive, is strongly influenced by profits.

This offensive viewpoint, when it dominates our view as it does today, blinds us to seeing the many defenses we have that protect us from invad-ing pollutants. Yet, these defenses play a significant role in protecting us. We know how these defenses work, we know how they are handicapped, and we know how to honor and support them to make them even stronger and more effective. If we promote and support our defenses, the other team will score less and we will have less problems in all of these areas. If we optimize our defense the other team will remain scoreless, which is our point.

In this book, we are going to focus on the respiratory tract, the source of URIs, allergies, asthma, and all of the other problems that begin in the back of the nose. And not only URIs, but lower respiratory infections as well because most pulmonary infections like pneumonia and bronchitis begin with bacteria that first colonize the nose and then break off and are aspirated into the lungs to cause problems there. Other lung diseases, like pulmonary fibrosis, originate in response to irritants that escape our nasal defenses and get into the lungs.

As well as the trachea that goes to the lungs, there are openings in the upper part of the nose into the sinuses; the Eustachian canal goes to the middle ear, and there are tear ducts leading to the eyes. All of these connected areas commonly get infected from bacteria living in the back of the nose. Honoring and supporting our nasal defenses means that all of these problems will not be there because the irritants and infecting agents will not be there.

This simple spray and following Mom's advice to keep your nose clean will help you to overcome allergies, asthma, sinus problems, middle ear infections, and even help your body to better cope with whatever bugs are in the air during cold and flu season. That's our argument in a nutshell: Keep your nose clean and you can get rid of these problems for good.

In the following chapters we will learn what our defenses are, how they are hobbled, and how we can help them to work better. And making them work better can keep us free of upper respiratory problems, infections included. We can live quite well without these problems.

CHAPTER TWO

The Discovery

I was exposed very early in my career as a doctor to the principle of oral rehydration and it framed a lot about my own view of medicine. The idea came from the success of drinking a sugar and salt solution to treat cholera in Bangladesh.

Cholera kills, not because of the infection per se, but because the body tries so vigorously to wash out the toxin the bacteria produce that we loose fluid too rapidly to replace. While cholera gets the blame, the cause of death is always dehydration.

Researchers found in the few years before I began practicing that a mixture of salt, sugar, and water was absorbed rapidly enough that one could keep enough fluid in the body for it to continue working despite the diarrhea. Hundreds of Bangladeshi women were trained to take this information to the people: a liter of water, a fist full of sugar, and a pinch of salt—and thousands of lives were saved. In 20 years oral rehydration saved more lives than penicillin had in 40, and the editors of the British medical journal *Lancet* called it one of the greatest achievements of 20th Century medicine.

We have learned since how it works and why it is so effective. The mixture of sugar and salt in the right proportions activates a pump in the stomach and small intestines that actively pumps water into the blood stream. It is by far the most effective and efficient way of getting water into the body that we have. But few people in this country know about it, a situation that leaders at Johns Hopkins called lamentable.

The reasons that so few know about oral rehydration are several: first of all salt and sugar are not patentable so this mixture cannot be a drug, even though it treats an illness effectively and saves thousands of lives. No drug status means no drug claims and no advertising; and in our society that translates to no one knowing. The second reason is the orientation of our health care system on profits. If a person presents with gastroenteritis to his local Emergency Department they will be treated with an IV, for which the hospital can bill in the range of $200, even if they are only mildly dehydrated and need only drink a few liters of oral rehydration, costing less than a quarter in Egyptian pharmacies, to get better.

The story and the success of oral rehydration played a large role in the way I practiced medicine. The most valuable information I regularly gave my patients was how to mix this up at home with a little more precision than the fist full of sugar approach. (You can read more in the Oral Rehydration section at the end of the book.) But it also convinced me that there may be other cures out there just waiting to be found that are equally effective. As it turns out the reason both oral rehydration and the nasal spray we developed are so successful is that both support a defense. But that is jumping the gun. Here's how the discovery unfolded.

EAR INFECTIONS AND SPECIAL EDUCATION

Jerry was trained in special education and much of her teaching career has been working with children who are not able to learn in the normal classroom. She knows that something bad happens when children, especially before age two, have recurrent ear infections. She knows this because when she asked her class, "Who has had tubes put in their ears?" everyone raised their hand. While Jerry knew there was a connection she didn't know why. What happens when ear infections become chronic is that the fluid secreted by the body to wash out infection tends to stay in the middle ear, and the middle ear is home to all of the small bones that carry the vibrations of the ear drum to the brain. Fluid from the middle ear dampens that transmission, so the pathways in the brain are not stimulated to become the myelinated roads and highways they should; and the pathways are destroyed in the pruning process that takes place at about age two. It is in this way that persistent inner ear fluid becomes a brain problem. Tubes are inserted into the eardrum in children with recurring ear infections in the attempt to reduce the fluid in the middle ear. This procedure sometimes helps to reduce the frequency of infections, but it is designed to help with hearing. Language, a critical part of early learning, is built by auditory input during the first two years of life, the same period when ear infections are most common. If this input is dampened by infection or fluid in the middle ear during this important period it takes persistent and determined effort on the part of parents and teachers to overcome the deficit. Dr. M. Luotonen and co-researchers demonstrated in the October 1996 issue of *Pediatric Infectious Disease Journal* that even when properly treated recurrent otitis during the first two years results in significant impairment in reading ability up to the age of nine. Dr. K.E. Bennett and co-researchers reported in the August 2001 issue of *Arch Dis Child* that they followed the children longer and showed significant learning and social problems extending up to age eighteen.

There are also now conditions like post otitis auditory disorder (POAD) or central auditory processing dysfunction (CAPD) that reflect and recognize some of the long-term problems associated with chronic ear infections, but most physicians have not made a connection; they see these as educational problems, not medical. These long-term studies indicate that tubes don't help much to reduce the educational problems that accompany chronic ear infections. If the problem is not dealt with the child can get frustrated with the educational process and often develops behavior problems.

There is not much that medicine can do when these infections become chronic. The British Health Service no longer treats patients with "glue ear"; doctors just give them pain medicine and wait for it to resolve on its own; antibiotics don't seem to help much. Despite their not working we in the United States often wait several months for a trial of antibiotics before placing the tubes, without even considering that this wait eliminates even more of the developmental window when learning sounds is optimal; when the pathways can still be myelinated and turned into roads. While these conditions are known they have not made it into our standard list of medical conditions. Ignored by the medical profession because they are not medical problems these long-term educational handicaps rob our children of optimal growth and functioning. Maybe now that we have a couple of acronyms for the condition the rest of the world will learn more about this connection.

As physicians we tend to ignore this problem of fluid in the middle ear; if there is no infection the fluid eventually does go away. In the meantime it contributes substantially to the population of children in our Special Education programs and to the expense that goes along with them. This educational expense is not even considered in the figures showing the costs of ear infections, but ear infections are one of the most common causes of Special Education services—and they are preventable. Jerry wouldn't let me ignore it. Today when we are talking about how prevention can help reduce medical costs we need to realize that the billions of dollars saved by reducing ear infections is eclipsed by the savings in our educational systems.

When Heather was put into day care so that her mother could return to teaching, she promptly began getting ear infections—four in the next five months.

The sense of urgency with which Jerry said, "You're a doctor, DO SOME-THING!" coincided with my reading about a Finnish chewing gum study in the November 9, 1996, issue of *The British Medical Journal*. The Finns knew about xylitol! They had used it for nearly forty years to prevent tooth decay. Now they showed that it prevented 42 percent of ear infections in a group, like Heather, that had recurrent problems.

Heather provided the *necessity* that fosters invention and this study showed the way.

But Heather was only eight months old, far too young to chew gum. The Finnish researchers said that the effect of xylitol was on the bacteria and those bacteria were in Heather's nose. I thought it prudent to put it there so I got some xylitol and had my hospital pharmacy mix it into a saline spray.

Mom and dad and day care workers sprayed her nose with one spray in each side every diaper change and the ear infections went away until they hired a new helper at day care that didn't know about the nose washing. She got an earache with that, but it responded to resuming the regular washing.

Three months later Heather's dad suggested that I get the spray patented, which I did. I also went to the Food and Drug Administration or FDA and told them I had a way to wash the nose. The FDA responded that they did not have a category for a nose wash and asked what cleaning your nose did. When I told them of my observations they said it was a drug.

Drugs are substances that prevent, treat or ameliorate a medical condition and this seemed to fit. A hundred years ago when the FDA was started there were arguments to include soap because it does this as well. But soap was considered a cosmetic and its benefits were secondary to its ability to clean the body. As we will see it's the same with xylitol, and if washing your hands is effective in reducing communicable diseases, washing the nose is even more so. Like soap xylitol is able to remove harmful bacteria from the nose; in addition it pulls more water into the nose to help with the washing. It is, in effect, soap for the nose; not a drug, but more like a cosmetic, just a simple natural way to wash your nose. And it is.

I mentioned that about a year later the local paper ran a story about Heather's ear infections. As a result I had a lot of parents come with their children from all over the state and some from other states. Their concerned grandparents, living in our town, told their children about Heather and how cleaning her nose stopped her ear infections. As I mentioned earlier, I saw these children one time so it can't be considered a proper scientific study, but it can tell about how these families used the health care system. About a year later I was able to contact ten of these families. Prior to washing their noses the parents of these children reported an average of 0.86 ear infections a month over the previous 5 months, with a doctor visit and an antibiotic prescription each time. Over an average of 11 months of washing the nose the ear complaints and doctor visits dropped to 0.06, which is a 92 percent decrease. In addition, of the seven ear infections that did occur, 3 were in one child and 3 occurred when use of the spray lapsed for a period of time. The way to treat ear infections is to prevent them and the way to prevent them is to wash the nose regularly.

The second child I used this with was JM. His mother was also a special education teacher. JM had already had two sets of ventilation tubes. After the second set came out the eardrum did not heal so he needed surgery to correct that. And he still had the condition called chronic suppurative otitis media, which is persistent fluid in the middle ear not associated with infection. This is the type of problem that eventually goes away as the child gets older. JM took longer and kept having problems. There is no treatment for this except waiting or putting in another set of tubes, but as noted above there is indication now that tubes do not really help the hearing and language problems that accompany this fluid. JM's mother was vigorous in spraying his nose. Three days later he gagged and vomited a huge amount of mucus at the dinner table, but he was better from that time on. The volume on the TV went down, he was better at discriminating word sounds, called phonemes, and the dark areas under his eyes went away. And two weeks later his auditory test for how well his ear drums were functioning, known a tympanogram, was normal.

From these first few cases, I knew that xylitol was something special. The Finnish research was suggesting that it was a sugar that bacteria in the body could not digest. It has only five carbon rings compared to the six that constitute the kinds of sugars, like glucose, that are the primary foods of bacteria that live with animals. Xylose, the source of xylitol, is plant sugar and while there are many bacteria that can easily handle it they aren't usually a problem to animals. Now the issue became how everything was linked together.

THE SINUS LINK

Well, sinus infections are similar to ear infections, and both Jerry and I used to have re-occurring sinus infections. I have used saline off and on for the past twenty years and found it to reduce the frequency of my infections a little. I began washing my nose with the xylitol and I had Jerry use saline. We were away at a conference when she got her last sinus infection; she was not happy being the control in our two-person study. Now she is using the xylitol spray in her nose too and we have both been free of any further sinus infections—more than 12 years and counting!

ATTACKING ALLERGIES

The first person who used this spray for allergies was my grandson Joe. He was allergic to grandmother's cat and they were due for a visit. My daughter called and asked what to do. I gave her all of the normal things to do to try to avoid exposure: shampoo the carpets, keep the cat outside, reserve a close motel room in case, and stock up on antihistamines. And I sent her a bottle of the spray. She used it about every four hours and Joe had no problems except when he first woke up after a night's rest when mom noticed some swelling around the eyes. This was gone about 30 minutes after the first spray. Dad took the kids back for another visit several months later and was there for about four hours when Joe's face started swelling. He called my daughter and asked her to "FedEx the spray." After a night elsewhere they were able to resume the visit with regular use of the spray. Joe, like many other children with allergies, has developed asthma and has an inhaler at home for bronchodilator treatments. He has begun washing his nose regularly and finds that three times a day, with more on occasion when he gets challenged, is enough to keep him clear. It was also enough to eliminate problems with grandma's cat during a recent visit.

The question you have is probably the same one I did: How can one simple spray (and it isn't even a drug) help with so many diverse health issues?

The answer has to do with our defenses. If our favorite football team has a real good defense it is very hard for their opponents to score; if we hobble their defense they will lose the game—and it's the same with us in our fight against the biological agents that cause these conditions.

Our body's defenses are the best available and they are concentrated where they can do the most good—in the areas of our body that are more open to infection:

• the airway where we exchange air;
• the gastrointestinal tract where we take in food and water;
• and the genitourinary tract, mostly the female genitourinary tract, that is open to sexually transmitted infections.

In this book, we are going to focus almost solely on how to help the defenses in the respiratory tract.* However, to a small extent, affecting this one area of health probably will portend good things for the rest of your body.

---

*Information on the other defenses and how to help them can be found in *The Boids and the Bees: Guiding Adaptation to Improve our Health, Healthcare, Schools, and Society.* The Institute for the Study of Coherence and Emergence. 2009.

THE NASAL CONNECTION

Keeping the nose clean with xylitol is important because essentially all respiratory problems have their beginning there. The back of the nose is connected to the middle ear by the Eustachian canal, the sinuses by the osteomeatal complex, and even to the eyes by the tear ducts. The nose is a nidus, a nest from which bacteria and viruses spread to other parts of the body. Allergens are first sensed there, and the bacteria and viruses that cause ear and sinus infections first attach there, and even the common cold and the flu come from viruses and bacteria that begin their journey in the back of the nose. All of these connected areas can get irritated by allergens or infected by viruses or bacteria that live in the back of the nose. Honoring and supporting our nasal defenses in their attempts to wash out these irritants means that these problems will cease. In the following we will show what our defenses are, how they are hobbled, and how we can help them work better. And making them work better can keep us free of upper respiratory problems, infections included.

After the FDA suggested that xylitol would be better classified as a drug because of its ability to stop ear and sinus infections and help with allergies and asthma, I began talking to drug companies to see if there was any interest in them jumping through regulatory hoops and marketing this spray. Initially there was, but it evaporated when they learned that the active ingredient, xylitol, was generally available and could not be protected by patent. The patent I got was a 'use' patent, meaning that no one could market the nasal use of xylitol. Drug companies want a patent either on the active ingredient, the drug itself, or on the medical device that delivers it. There are also other ways of defining drugs, like if they are taken internally. This is the problem we share with oral rehydration; both have sufficient benefit to be classed as "drugs," but neither have the ability to reward the drug companies with sufficient profits to make that practical. Again: no patent—no profits; no profits—no research; no research—and no one knows about the benefits. There is no economical way that a common safe food substance can be a 'drug' so this spray is not regulated or approved by the FDA. It is not a drug; it is only a very neat way to wash your nose. If washing your hands is effective in reducing communicable diseases, washing the nose is even more so because that is where so many of them enter the body.

Yet research done on nasally administered xylitol satisfies the most demanding standards: it acts locally and is not absorbed into the nasal tissues; that means that it winds up in our stomachs just like the xylitol we eat in berries or other fruits. In addressing the safety of this spray for the FDA I wrote: "Ten percent of the dry weight of a plum is xylitol. If a person were to use this spray every hour of the day, 24 hours a day, both sides of the nose, they would get the equivalent of half a plum's worth of xylitol." When I withdrew my application for consideration at the FDA they remarked on the impressive safety profile.

XYLITOL—THE BACK STORY

Technically xylitol is the sugar alcohol of xylose, which is wood sugar. But that is misleading because xylitol is neither a sugar, nor an alcohol. It looks like sugar and it tastes like sugar, but it has very little effect on a person's blood sugar and is metabolized in an entirely separate way from the other sugars we eat.

Xylose, wood sugar, is actually a very common sugar in the human body. It is one of the seven sugar complexes on our cell surfaces that are used by the cells to recognize one another. It is by means of these sugar complexes that our cells hold on to each other and know where to hold on. It is also these sugar complexes that bacteria attach to. Most of the sugars we use for energy are six carbon sugars like glucose and fructose, and some of them have unfamiliar names, like galactose, mannose, and fucose. Xylose and xylitol only have five carbons and xylitol also differs from the others in that it is flexible. In the body the six carbon sugars are generally fixed in their shape; they are in a ring form that can bind easily and regularly with other sugars to form chains of simple sugars, and they are stable enough that other cells and bacteria looking for something to hold on to can rely on them not to change. Xylose is also commonly in a ring formation, but xylitol is only open. This means that it is flexible; it can bend and twist and look like a lot of these other receptors; in other words, it can fill up the hands the bacteria use to hold on. I think this is significant to how xylitol works and will talk more about it later.

Another reason for it to work is suggested from the early dental studies; xylitol gives the bacteria indigestion—they eat it, but they can't digest it.

Was the same thing happening in the nose? I called Dr. Matti Uhari in Finland and told him of my experience. Dr. Uhari is one of the world's leading xylitol researchers; it was his study that showed what chewing xylitol-sweetened gum could do for preventing ear infections. He thought I should try to reproduce his studies with the chewing gum. That didn't make much sense because his study prevented only 42 percent of ear infections using gum that cost about a dollar a day; the spray prevented about 92 percent of infections at a cost of about 7 cents a day. I suggested that he reproduce mine, but he wasn't interested.

Dr. Uhari did tell me about a study his group had done that was due to be published. In this study they showed that xylitol blocked much of the bacteria's ability to hold on to the cells in our noses. We will also talk more about this study a little later, but it is a major part of this story because it shows that the action is not just bacterial indigestion.

CHAPTER THREE

The Importance of Your Nasal Defenses

The spectrum of problems we term Upper Respiratory Infections are the most common presenting complaints to primary care physicians, and they all start in the back of the nose. This may be repetitious, but it's important. Beginning from their home in the back of the nose, bacteria move down the Eustachian canal to cause otitis media in children, climb up through the ostiomeatal complex to cause sinus infections in older people, and, while properly termed lower respiratory infections, bacteria and viruses that are able to get airborne in the nose get aspirated to cause bronchitis and pneumonia. The major pathogen in the nose, *Streptococcus pneumoniae*, is responsible for the deaths of about 40,000 Americans every year and over a million deaths worldwide, but this particular bacteria, and its family, turns out to be particularly susceptible to xylitol.

Upper respiratory conditions are a major cause of loss time at work and they have many associated problems even after we recover from the acute illness. Furthermore the treatment of these conditions is the primary reason for the use of antibiotics, often even when antibiotics are likely to be modestly if at all helpful; and the over-utilization of these antibiotics is the primary source of antibiotic resistance. Upper respiratory conditions are a major problem, both for the illnesses they cause, the effects of those illnesses, and the response the antibiotics used to treat them provoke in our bacteria.

Also, the problem is likely to worsen.

These days, studies are now showing that along with rising sea levels, melting icecaps and stronger hurricanes, allergies are also increasing.

Findings by Harvard Environmental Science and Engineering research associate Christine Rogers indicate there may be a whole lot more sneezing, sniffling, and scratching in the next few years—all thanks to global warming.

She says that levels of carbon dioxide could increase from 350 parts per million in the atmosphere to as much as 700 ppm, spurring the growth of more ragweed and opportunistic plants. Ragweed is a prime producer of pollen.

"There have been significant increases in allergies and asthma in recent decades, which obviously cannot be explained by any change in genetics," she said.

In 2005 some 40 million Americans suffered from hay fever. Another 16 million adults endured asthma with rates markedly increasing among inner city youth, particularly as a result of urban pollution and increasing pollen counts due to global warming.

Rogers found plant flowering times and airborne pollen concentrations are changing. Global warming is increasing photosynthesis and more plant growth.

"Plants are flowering significantly earlier over time and advancing the season by approximately 0.8 days per year," Rogers said.

Other research has found increasing plant growth in Arctic lakes and that total seasonal pollen production per plant has increased.

Rogers said that global warming is causing aeroallergens to be abundant and they are causing newly allergic people to have stronger more frequent symptoms.

Dealing with these problems costs tens of billions of dollars every year in health care costs, but their social costs are often far greater. The cost of educating a normal child is far less than what it costs to educate a child with a learning difficulty, like children with POAD, or CAPD; and allergies play a role here as well. But while they are caused by medical conditions these educational costs are not included in the medical costs.

Take this recent study I came across. Done in the Netherlands and reported in the *Annals of Allergy* the researchers looked at children in a classroom situation. Included were normal children as well as those with allergies. Those with allergies were divided into three groups: the first was treated with a placebo, that supposedly has no medical effect; the second with a sedating antihistamine, like Benadryl®; and the third with a non-sedating antihistamine, like Claritin®. Then they looked at how well these children learned. All of the children with allergies did worse than the those without them; the allergy condition itself distracts from optimal learning. Worst off were those treated with the placebo and sedating antihistamine, but even the non-sedating antihistamine adversely affected learning.

While Xylitol is not by any means regulated as a drug like these medications, its use in this case would be to support your child's health and help to maintain already healthy nasal tissues with regular washing. Now that's simple.

I mentioned that our primary means of coping with upper respiratory infections is prescribing an antibiotic. Antibiotics kill the invading organism and most of the time the person suffering gets better. But we know now that antibiotics don't do much when these infections become chronic. We also know that the bacteria in our gut are often killed as well, and they are the ones that help us digest our food, make vitamins and other substances that we need in order to live, and are part of our primary gastrointestinal defense system. And when antibiotics threaten these GI bacteria they develop resistance.

Every living organism has some ability to read its environment and adapt to it, but few do it as speedily as bacteria. We know, for example, that bacteria increase their mutation rate when they are threatened, and that if enough of them participate in this mutation, a solution to the threat is not far off. Unlike us, however, where we would patent and profit from such a genetic adaptation, these bacteria give it away freely not only to family and friends, but to any bacteria interested. So now we have antibiotic resistant bacteria out in our communities and around the world.

So far our response to this threat has been to rely on ever more powerful antibiotics, which kill more bacteria, but also stimulate more resistance. We are engaged in an arms race with bacteria, a race that for several reasons we have little chance of winning.

First of all bacteria are the most persisting of species; by any measure, "length of dominion, prospects for survival, tenacity, sheer abundance, genetic or biochemical diversity, or range of current habitats" bacteria come out on top—they are the titans of life on earth. Another handicap we have is the nature of this race; pharmaceutical companies are tremendously handicapped. In order to develop a new antibiotic there needs to be the following elements, as I learned in my own experience when I offered up my very effective nasal xylitol: a patent to insure that the company can make a profit; lots of expensive research (they need to test on animals first—and because of animal testing some of the new antibiotics already have resistant bacteria by the time they are released for human use); and they need patients or insurance companies who can pay for them to support more research. This process takes years.

On the other hand, the development of resistance in bacteria is much faster. Stressed bacteria, like those living in our gastrointestinal or GI tracts where they get a full dose of our antibiotics, can increase their mutation rate by more than 1000 times. Not all of them do this because if they all started mutating it would be suicidal. Mutation is a random process and leads to more problems than successes, but there are enough bacteria mutating that resistance comes relatively rapidly. The resistant mutation is then shared vertically by these bacteria multiplying, and multiplying unopposed since the antibiotic has cleared many of the competitors from the field; and it is shared laterally with other bacteria, even unrelated bacteria, by a variety of means including small capsules called plasmids, kind of a viral prototype, with no concern at all for intellectual property rights or a profit. They are a formidable foe and we have little chance of winning this war.

A realistic look at the past shows us our odds in this warfare. Bacteria were the first forms of life on our planet. For about two billion years they were the only life. They formed the atmosphere we breathe. They learned to recycle themselves and other organic material. Some of them learned to use the energy from sunlight and others learned to make it from sugars. About a billion and a half years ago some of these bacteria, maybe just two, cooperated and gave up their individual lives to be a part of a larger cell. The bacteria that knew how to make energy from sugars became the mitochondria that supply the energy for all cells, and the bacteria that had learned how to use sunlight became the chloroplasts that are in all plant cells. Millions of different life forms came from that cooperative beginning, but now, a billion and a half years later, more than 95 percent of these advanced life forms are extinct. On the other hand 99 percent of the bacteria living at that time are still around. Those are not very good odds when one is choosing sides in a war.

Like our battle with 'terrorism' this is seen as a 'cosmic war,' a battle between the forces of good and those of evil, and the only way to win a cosmic war, points out Reza Aslan, in his book *How to Win a Cosmic War*, is not to fight one. In our warfare with bacteria this means, as countless infectious disease specialists repeatedly point out, that we need to control our use of antibiotics. But these scientists have no plan on how to do so; and they may be dragging their feet because denouncing the war while letting it proceed is far more profitable.

You and I are different. We are going to make our own health. We have a plan! Keep your nose clean with xylitol!

A COUNTRY DOCTOR'S VIEW

Not only does our health care system not have a workable plan to deal with antibiotic resistance, but the incidence of upper respiratory problems has been increasing over the past forty years. Some feel that part of the reason for this is our system. In a provocative article titled "Is U.S. health really the best in the world?" published in the July 26, 2000, issue of *The Journal of the American Medical Association* Barbara Starfield, MD, MPH, of the Johns Hopkins Bloomberg School of Medicine offers up facts that show that our health care system is the third leading cause of death in this country, behind heart disease and cancer. In pointing this out, the public health policy expert looked mostly at our hospital infections, our surgical errors, and the complications of our drugs. She did not look at the effect of our drugs in turning off many of our more uncomfortable defenses. This was not considered a problem, but it makes our system even more dangerous. The doctor, for example, did not look at the recent withdrawal of cold and cough medicines for children that came from the finding that several children had died following the use of these readily available drugs. While the FDA and pharmaceutical industry blame overuse of the drugs by parents, which compounded their side effects, no one sees the simple connection that these drugs block a helpful defense, and that blocking a defense eliminates its survival benefit. Eliminating a survival benefit means more people will die; and that is what happened.

There is also an interesting correlation between the use of these drugs and increases in upper respiratory problems. Side effect studies for these drugs are done before the FDA will allow them to be released, but the studies look only at the side effects for taking the drug, like sedation, sleep disturbance, nausea, or dry nose, for antihistamines. Few of them ask the question that really matters: what the drug does to life expectancy. They usually last about two weeks, which is normally long enough to see the side effects, but nowhere near long enough to see the long-term results of taking the drugs. In the case of the cough and cold pills it took about 60 years for the FDA to see a connection between their use and deaths among children. That's actually an improvement; it took close to three thousand for doctors to see a connection between bloodletting and more people dying. And I may be a bit generous because the FDA still thinks the problem is parental overdosing and not the results of hobbling a useful defense.

Of course, one of our most prevalent allergy, cold, flu and sinus medication families are the antihistamines, which inhibit the body's production of histamine. There were earlier hints pointing to the dangers of antihistamines, but they were not seen because we were asking the wrong questions. Until around 2001 *The Physicians' Desk Reference*, the big red or blue reference book that tells doctors about the drugs they prescribe, reported on the side effect studies for the drug loratadine (Claritin®), one of the new "non-sedating" antihistamines. This study can still be found at a variety of drug sites on the Internet. The side effect studies for this and other drugs, again, look only at the side effects; they do not look at the long-term effects of taking the drugs. They generally last about two weeks, and the ones for antihistamines and cold medicines are usually done in the summer when the infectious problems associated with the nose are less prevalent. Because of this timing the number of children with problems never got high enough to be significant, but the study of loratadine showed a doubling of both URIs and wheezing during its two-week course. If this study had been done in the winter 'cold season' when a fourth or a third of the students are commonly out with colds, and the same doubling held, we would not likely have this drug.

In 1992, the National Center for Health Statistics published data showing the increases in otitis between 1975, when there were 10 million cases, and

1990 when there were 25 million. Ear infections have been increasing at a rate of about 5 percent per year ever since the early 1970s, and so have sinus infections according to the ear, nose and throat doctors. Infectious disease specialists have tried to find reasons for the increases in otitis and look mostly at day care and the sharing of germs there that most are at a loss to control. Try as best they can workers in these centers cannot keep up with the children as they share their toys during play along with all of the bacterial and viral contents of their runny noses. Within days a new bacteria generally spreads to every child in a center. They are recognized in the health care industry as social cesspools. Sometimes our work places are almost as bad.

The data for asthma also show regular increases, but the underlying reasons are accepted as being more complex. Left out of this complexity, however, is any sense that it may be the fault of the system. A recent observation adding to the complexity is that the asthma increases seen in the west are not seen in eastern bloc countries such as Russia and Albania.

The most complete information on the increases in asthma from the whole country comes from the Centers for Disease Control and Prevention (CDC) where they have collected information on asthma prevalence since the 1980s. This data is represented in Figure 1.

Figure 1

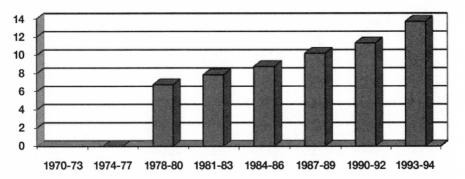

Self Reported Asthma in Millions

Figure 1–Mannino, et al. MMWR CDC Surveill Summ 4/24/1998.
Data taken from their Table 1.

More telling is data on hospital admissions for asthma collected by researchers at the Medical University of South Carolina in Charleston. They reported hospital admissions for asthma by race going back to 1956, represented in Figure 2. The authors of this study, seeing the stable baseline that extended throughout the 60s, tried to find a reason for the increases that began in the 70s. They looked at changes in pollution, new industries, and changes in plant pollens; following the pattern of western medicine they looked at all of the things that were outside of the patient—and they could not find anything. They finally looked at the parallel increases in obesity during that time period and concluded there must be a connection. What they failed to see was the correlation with the drugs we now know cause more deaths in children.

Figure 2

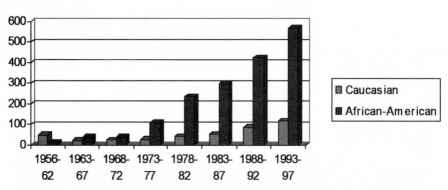

Crater DD, Heise S, Perzanowski M, Herbert R, Morse CG, Hulsey TC, Platts-Mills T. "Asthma hospitalization trends in Charleston, South Carolina, 1956 to 1997: twenty-fold increase among black children during a 30-year period." *Pediatrics* 2001 Dec; 108(6): E97.

Cough and cold medicines, the ones withdrawn from use for children in the fall of 2007, are mostly antihistamine and decongestant combinations. They were the miracle drugs of the 1940s. We had learned in the 1930s that histamine was the cause of Johnny's runny nose, and in the 1940s we developed antihistamines that stopped it. It was a wonderful advance because we could now give our children with this problem a dose of medicine and take them to day care and not have to miss a day of work. But a runny nose, rhinorrhea in medical terms, is there to wash the irritant out of the nose. That's common sense; our nose doesn't run except when it is irritated. But what happens when we turn off this defense by using cough and cold medicines? Blocking the runny nose with loratadine doubled both the rate of URIs and the incidence of wheezing, and their comparison study with one of the older 'sedating' antihistamines showed it to cause even more wheezing. Are the results from the Charleston study related to what these drugs do? Many biologists are beginning to see this connection.

The 1970s saw several things happen that greatly enhanced these drugs' use. First of all they were deemed safe enough by the FDA to be made available without a prescription. Second, the wide use of television provided an optimal means for the pharmaceutical companies to market them; and third, the advent of Medicaid provided a means to get them into the hands of our poorer populations. But this connection is circumstantial; it is not enough for proof. In my university logic class I learned that *'after this, therefore because of this'* was not a logical argument, and this fits that pattern. If that were all there was it would not hold any water. To see how the use of these drugs contributes to upper respiratory problems we have to understand what goes on in the airway when allergens and infectious agents threaten it; and this requires that we see the problem differently. First we will look at allergies and asthma, then the infectious problem.

ALLERGIES AND ASTHMA

What is asthma? The traditional and leading definition is inflammation of the airway that leads to both its acute and chronic constriction. But that is just a problem oriented definition; it defines the condition in terms of the symptoms without any consideration for what is going on that leads to the symptoms.

Most people think of asthma as not being able to breathe. The muscles that surround our bronchial tubes go into spasm, shutting down the airway and causing this suffocating feeling. Our efforts to cope with asthma have focused on this spasm and found drugs that help these muscles relax and not be so trigger-happy in the first place. We know several things from our scientific and clinical studies with asthma:

- It is caused by the immune system.
- The major mechanism is through the nasal-bronchial reflex where irritants in the back of the nose lead to the broncho-constriction we know as asthma.
- Medical researchers have analyzed the mechanism behind the nasal-bronchial reflex and developed a variety of drugs that modify this reflex. We have bronchodilators that reverse the broncho-constriction; and *when someone is having an asthma attack we need to use these drugs.* They save lives. We also have drugs to prevent asthma: leukotriene antagonists and inhibitors that interfere with a part of this reflex, and steroids that turn much of it off.

But let's take another step back and look at what is going on here. When we do this we are in new territory because our healthcare system is stuck on the *how*; seldom do they ask *why*. Once we see that cleaning the nose resolves asthma we have to ask how and why; and the following conclusions become common sense.

First of all the immune system is designed to keep us healthy, and while it can occasionally cause problems for us, in all fairness, it does this primarily, even when it kills us (as it does with cholera and asthma), to protect us from what it considers a greater danger. Reflexes in the body are generally there to protect us. Our pupillary *reflex* closes the eye and protects it from too much light, and our gag *reflex* protects us from aspirating food. The nasal-bronchial reflex that triggers asthma protects our lungs from the pollutants in our nose.

A story from Miami may be illustrative: Dr. Copeland was the medical examiner in Dade County Florida. He did a series of autopsies on people who had drowned and found that about 20 percent of these people had dry lungs. Before this study was done bodies found in the water with dry lungs were presumed to have been killed elsewhere then dumped into the water, but Dr. Copeland's subjects were known to have drowned. The coroner's conclusion was that the water in their nose prompted such a profound laryngeal and bronchospasm that they could not breathe in the water. This spasm is the same thing we see in asthma, so these people died of an asthma attack. That is, their immune systems, recognizing that the water in their upper airway would kill them if it got into their lungs shut down their airway to prevent that from happening

Asthma, in this new way of seeing it, is a defense, and while we need to take the drugs that enable us to breathe when we can't, we also need to see the value of just cleaning out what our immune systems are so afraid of. I was just beginning to look at a group of children with asthma when my local hospital and clinic folded. Try as I might I could never convince any one else to pick up this study. Picking up someone else's research is not easy, but neither is seeing our problems with new eyes.

INFECTIOUS PROBLEMS IN THE NOSE

Aside from allergies, the second most common trigger for asthma is a respiratory infection. Respiratory syncytial virus is a particularly common trigger for asthma in children, and so are sinus infections, as Traci's case in our introduction illustrates.

The major bacterial agent causing URIs is *Streptococcus pneumoniae*, a lethal bacteria, discussed earlier, that kills over a million people worldwide every year. 'Strep', as it is commonly called, kills mostly when it gets into the brain, but it causes major problems in the lungs, joints, and in the belly. All these infections begin when this bacteria is allowed to live in the back of the nose; and this is common. The nose is where these bacteria hang out in humans; it is their reservoir.

It is common enough that our pharmaceutical industry developed an immunization to help us recognize and deal with several members of this family of bacteria that caused most of the infections. Most tactical maneuvers have initial success until the enemy figures them out and develops an effective response, and this was no exception. While this immunization closed the doorway to the targeted strains it just opened it for others. Infections from the targeted strains did drop, but the other strains are picking up on the opportunity and are becoming more virulent. All living agents, including simple bacteria, adapt to changes in their environment and when they are threatened they adapt by developing resistance and becoming stronger; as Nietzsche said, "What doesn't kill me makes me stronger," and it's not just people that do this, it's all living things. We need to be more careful in how we deal with living agents around us including bacteria.

Pasteur spent most of his life studying the microbes that infect us, but there is another side to infection—the host and their defenses. Pasteur's counter in this argument was Claude Bernard and there is a story, that is most likely apocryphal, that Pasteur honored Bernard on his deathbed by acknowledging that the soil, or the terrain, was more important than the seed. The truth is it takes two to tango and the seed and the soil both play important parts, but our researchers have more often than not followed Pasteur and neglected the defenses we all have that make up the other part of this dance. We need to look more at host factors and the part they play in why we get sick; and we need to find ways to help correct or compensate for the ones that weaken us and support those that help us. Children, whose immune systems are not well formed yet, and the elderly, whose immune systems are hampered by age, are more at risk. Even more so are those with immune deficiencies or those who have had their spleens removed for trauma or other reasons. Even pregnancy with the changes to the immune system it demands, seems to weaken our defenses to the flu. These host factors hamper our immune system's ability to recognize and cope with these problematic bacteria.

And there are a whole lot of other bacteria that work like Strep. *Neisseria meningitidis*, the bacteria that cause epidemic meningitis, first colonize the back of the nose. So do the strains of *Haemophilus influenzae* that, until the immunization for these bacteria was developed, was a major culprit in childhood meningitis.

Sometimes infections don't have to begin in the nose. When a person has allergies and persistent nasal congestion they have to breathe through their mouth. This bypasses all of the nasal defenses and allows more viruses and bacteria to get directly into the lungs where the defenses are not nearly as robust. As well as helping and supporting our nose's defenses we need to keep it open so that we don't bypass its protection by mouth breathing.

Even when these infections don't kill they can result in many other problems. Hearing and seizure problems are common in those who are fortunate enough to survive infections in the brain, and arthritis commonly follows joint infections; and we have already looked at the educational problems that follow chronic ear infections.

A CLOSER LOOK AT MIDDLE EAR INFECTIONS

Middle ear infections are the most common URI in children, but many are confused about them. Some seem to think that putting medication in the ear can treat them and I have even met doctors who were unsure about how the bacteria get into the middle ear space. The Eustachian canal connects the back of the nose with the middle ear, the space behind the eardrum; it's the tube that allows the air pressure to equalize on both sides of the ear drum as we drive into the mountains or dive into the seas, and it lets bacteria move from the back of the nose into the middle ear. These infections are the overwhelming reason for the use of antibiotics in children, but this use, along with other cases of overuse, is developing its own set of problems since it stimulates the development of antibiotic resistance in the bacteria exposed to them. These resistant bacteria develop into super-bugs that we cannot kill with antibiotics. Because of this specialists dealing with infectious diseases are encouraging doctors to be more judicious in their use of antibiotics; but we need more than just being judicious. We desperately need a different way to look at and deal with this problem. This is what we propose; that is what keeping your nose clean is all about.

In the days before antibiotics adequate treatment for most ear infections was lancing the eardrum with a small knife and allowing the infection to drain. But antibiotics were just as effective early on, a lot simpler, a lot less traumatic, and they prevented the complication of meningitis that occurred when bacteria got into the porous bones around the middle ear and from there into the brain. Antibiotics were a better choice then because they killed these bacteria. But that was before we saw the problem of antibiotic resistance, before we realized we were in a cosmic war with bacteria, and engaged in an arms race where the antibiotic treatment of ear infections plays a major role in stimulating resistance and escalating the war. While this role is recognized by most, few deal it with because we have not seen other options.

WHY ANTIBIOTICS DON'T WORK
WELL ENOUGH ANYMORE

When antibiotics were first developed they were very effective. The dose of amoxicillin needed to treat an ear infection was about 250 milligrams a day for ten days; it's now close to ten times that. Back then we also knew very little about the role bacteria play in the workings of our bodies. We know a lot more now. We know that good bacteria help us live by providing many of the nutrients we need and that they play a critical role in many of our primary defenses by providing a shield against bad bacteria.

Several years ago my wife and I visited the Great Barrier Reef off the east coast of Australia. We were cautioned, before we dove, against touching any of the reef or animals because they were protected by a biofilm, a film made up of friendly bacteria that protected these animals from other agents, viruses or bacteria, which could infect them. Touching them could potentially remove this biofilm and open them to infection.

We have the same protective elements working in our bodies; good bacteria live in our noses, our gastrointestinal tracts, and our genitourinary tracts, and on our skin, where they help protect us against many bacteria from outside by robbing them of places to hold on as well as food to eat. We know, for example, that women who douche regularly open themselves to different bacteria that are not as protective against a variety of infections, from bacterial vaginosis to HIV. The same holds true for disturbing the friendly bacteria in our noses or GI tracts when we take antibiotics. In a way this kind of protection even extends outward as our immune systems get used to those bacteria in our environment. Women considering home birthing, for example, are cautioned about the increased possibility of infection if they have not lived in their home for a few months—long enough to get familiar with the bacteria that are present.

While our pharmaceutical companies try to make antibiotics that are selective and don't kill the good bacteria this is largely an effort in futility since there is DNA evidence of hundreds of bacteria in our GI tracts that we have not even identified, let alone added to the list of health friendly species, and it is the bacteria in our GI tracts that are mostly those developing resistance.

And it's not just our GI tract bacteria doing this; animals participate on an even greater scale. In 1954 we made 2 million pounds of antibiotics and now we make over 50 million. More than 70 percent of antibiotic production goes to animals where it stimulates the growth of resistance just as it does in humans. Antibiotics are used in animals to prevent epidemics in their unhealthy massive feeding lots, but most use is because antibiotics have been found to promote growth—and this part is totally unregulated. Better feed, probiotics, and a cleaner, more natural environment are safer and more effective ways of reducing infections, both in animals and humans.

We need another way to think about this problem. I am by no means saying never to use these powerful tools; they save lives. But most doctors routinely overprescribe them for many minor or viral infections where they do little good. If we ourselves can get by without taking antibiotics, the friendly ones will continue to help us live healthier lives; and if we as a society can use antibiotics more responsibly we will have less of a problem with resistant bacteria.

Early on antibiotic resistance was limited to hospitals where antibiotic use was more prevalent and higher dosages were used. But resistant bacteria are now spread around the world and everyone, even a healthy young person, is open to infection by these superbugs. They are a major problem in infectious disease that we need to resolve, and the way to resolve it is to rely less on our offensive team (antibiotics) and more on strengthening our defenses. That's one of the most important things I learned in my osteopathic training.

In our warfare with bacteria we have concentrated on the offensive. We have focused on the bacteria and viruses, searching for ways to kill them or help our bodies kill them. Yet we know now that this is neither practical nor possible—it isn't even desirable when we remember what the many good bacteria living with us do. Instead of concentrating on the offensive we need to remember the part our body's defenses play in this process. We need to remember that there are two sides in this dance, both the seed and the soil, and that we and our defenses are the soil.

Empowering defenses is not a one-time effort; it is creating a habit, like regularly washing your hands, that enhances health. Let me relate a few examples. We have already met JM whose chronic ear infections led to two sets of tubes and surgery to repair a non-closing eardrum. JM was adopted and he had several siblings who were also adopted; and like him they all had medical problems. His mom, like Mother Theresa, had a soft spot for kids with problems who would otherwise have been abandoned. Because she was busy with all of her special children she could not spend the time herself to make sure that JM used the spray regularly. When she stopped assisting and monitoring his use, JM's hearing problems returned and Mom had to rededicate herself to JM's regular nasal hygiene routine; and the embarrassing and messy coughing up of copious mucus occurred two more times in that year. The spray doesn't cure conditions; it just prevents problems; but to do this it has to be used regularly.

Traci, the young girl with asthma, demonstrates the same problem. Even though she was able to participate in sports and live free of asthma for several years she stopped using the spray regularly and her asthma did return. It's *keeping your nose clean using xylitol* that works and that means regular use. Children are not usually reliable at this; you have to help them.

Over the years we have found several ways to help in this process:

- Start early; the spray was designed for a baby and they generally adapt well to its use. Hold the baby upright and spray each nostril, then lay them down and change their diaper so the spray can move to the back of the nose where it is effective.

- Older children get to be resistant; they don't like others doing things to them, they want to be in control of themselves. But this can usually be negotiated; give them a choice whenever possible, like which side first. When we approach our grandson with the spray he will hold his nose closed and open his mouth. After a spray in his mouth he will open one side of his nose and allow us to spray there. Then we repeat the process for the other side. The spray is sweet and has a pleasant taste, and if you don't keep it out of their reach many small children will drink it. This doesn't hurt them, but it is not free and it's much more effective if it is passed through the nose than the mouth on the way to the stomach.

- By far the best way to promote its use is for everyone in the household to use it regularly; children learn by example so if you want them to keep their noses clean you better set a good example. Chewing gum studies show an optimal benefit preventing 80 percent of tooth decay when used five times a day; we argue the same for nasal use. If you or your kids are sick use the spray often, but as your health recovers, five times a day is fine if you have a chronic problem like allergies, even less often if you are normally healthy, but regular use daily is important. The advice I give to people worried about the flu is appropriate: When you wash your hands wash your nose, and drink enough water. Make sure that happens at least five times a day. I also realize this is ideal and that most people just will not use it that often. People seem to use it when they think about it, i.e. when they start to have a problem. But that may be too late. Take a good look at yourself and your environment. If you are generally healthy and don't have allergies you can likely get away with two to three times a day, but if you have a nasal-related condition or are exposed to a wide variety of infectious agents (like if you are a doctor, teacher, or a day care worker) then you had better find a way to use it more often, and the best way to do that is to associate washing your nose with something you do regularly.

BIOFILM AND INFECTIONS

Both Traci and JM (case 2 and 15) share another aspect of this story the bears looking at before leaving this subject. They both had episodes where they got rid of a bunch of foreign material in the back of their noses that was associated with their immediate improvement. What's going on here?

I wasn't there and they didn't bring any of this stuff for me to look at so this is mostly conjecture on my part, but it makes sense. We have already talked about biofilm and how it protects us and other animals. But there is also a down side. All bacteria can make biofilm; it's not just the friendly ones. When bad bacteria build biofilm it becomes a safe house for them to hide in and they are very difficult to remove; it takes doses of antibiotics a hundred times normal to reach bacteria in their safe houses, and that is enough to kill the person. We don't know very much about the role of biofilm in illness and the National Institutes of Health, which funds most health care research, won't even pay for biofilm research for this reason. But there is nevertheless a fair amount of research.

We know, first of all, how biofilm is formed. When bacteria get into the body the first thing they must do is find a place to hold on. If they can't hold on they are just washed out by the fluids bathing our bodies and we have no problem. If they find a way to hold on and are not recognized by our immune systems early on they multiply. As they increase in number they make a chemical that acts as a signal when it reaches a certain concentration. The process is called quorum sensing and it triggers some of the bacteria to start making biofilm—some, but not all. Just as in the case of bacteria mutating to find a means of coping with an antibiotic, for all of them to begin building a biofilm would be suicidal. People studying this process with powerful microscopes describe biofilm in terms reminiscent of a *Star Wars* city. You can see some of their pictures online at the web page hosted by the Center for Biofilm Engineering at the University of Montana. (See www.erc.montana.edu/cbessentials.) These bacterial homes are what protect the marine life as well as us when they are made up of helpful bacteria. When they are made up of harmful bacteria they cause long-term problems like chronic infections because the bacteria can stay inside their safe houses where the antibiotics can't reach them; ear infections are a perfect example.

We were recently visiting our foster son in Sweden and Jerry got involved talking with one of his friends, a medical student, about her favorite subject of ear infections. In Sweden, he explained, they find that viruses cause most chronic ear infections so they don't use antibiotics to treat them. She tried to explain the concept of biofilm to him, but it was new and unfamiliar, and he wasn't receptive. I wasn't there to lend her support, but what he was relying on are the studies where they take fluid from the middle ear of children with chronic ear infections and culture it to look for bacteria, and often they don't find any. It is easy to conclude from these studies that bacteria are not there so the infections must be viral, but that conclusion leaves out some significant information.

When fluid is taken from acutely infected middle ears the most common finding is both bacteria and viruses, and this is true for one-time infections or acute flare-ups in those with chronic otitis. And often the bacteria found in the acute flares of chronically infected ears are the same strain, which suggests that these recurrent infections may actually be the same infection. If fluid from these ears is cultured in between acute infections nothing is found, supporting what the Swedish medical student was arguing. But what if the bacteria causing these flares are just hiding out in their biofilm safe houses and are not exposed to the antibiotic used to treat the acute infections? This was a question asked by a group at Pittsburg who used DNA marking as a means of detecting bacterial biofilm. This test was positive 100 percent of the time when the middle ear fluid from children with chronic ear infections was examined, and 92 percent of the time when they looked at specimens of the middle ear surface membranes. While I was not there and the material they coughed and vomited up was not examined, I believe the cleansing episodes Traci and JM experienced were likely caused by the breaking loose of their biofilm.

I was thinking about this problem several years ago when I heard Randy Wolcott, one of our local doctors, talk about his work helping wounds to heal. Biofilm is a major problem because it always grows over open wounds and hampers healing. Dr. Wolcott was dealing with wounds of people with insufficient blood supply due to hardening of the arteries or diabetes; if he could not get the wounds to heal the treatment was generally amputation of the limb with the problem.

After his presentation I talked with him about my ideas with xylitol and bacterial adherence and he began experimenting on his own. The best results on getting these wounds to heal had been in the 65 percent range. Over the subsequent years he found that he could heal 77 percent of these wounds using a dressing containing significant amounts of xylitol and another naturally occurring antibiotic substance called lactoferrin. His nurses, the ones that took care of the wounds, told him that the wounds where the accumulated material at the wound surface would just come off with the dressing always healed. The Center for Biofilm Engineering at the University of Montana participated in this study and their director, Garth James, told me that their experiments showed that xylitol has a broad-spectrum ability to block biofilm formation and adherence. This has since been confirmed by Dr. Wolcott and a group working in Lubbock. Using a wound model with many different types of bacteria, they showed that a 20 percent solution of xylitol stopped all biofilm formation. So now I feel a lot more comfortable thinking that this is what happened with these two children.

Both good and bad bacteria build biofilm after they first find a way to hold on and are able to multiply. They have many ways to protect themselves and to adapt to their environments so that they can continue recycling the world. Recycling the world is what they have done for billions of years. They are not going to stop. Nor should we try to persuade them to. Life on earth would be intolerable without the bacteria recycling it. The problems of infectious disease all stem from their time honored function and ability to recycle us. It argues for fighting the bacteria, but at the same time we desperately need to realize the nature of the symbiotic relationship we have with our friendly bacteria; we could not live without them—or even without those that recycle us. We need to find another way to persuade them not to attack us while we are still alive; this will be the subject of a later chapter. And we need to find a way to keep our kids out of Special Education. Avoiding putting tubes in children's ears would certainly save us some serious medical treatment dollars. In order to do this we need to understand the nature of our nasal defenses and how to support them.

CHAPTER FOUR

Eliminating Asthma

In most areas of the body there are levels of defense and the nose is no exception. Our primary defenses, like the bacteria, acid, and enzymes in our stomachs and intestines, work without our noticing—until something goes wrong. When our GI defenses get overwhelmed the back up is gastroenteritis, nausea, vomiting, or diarrhea. Similarly the primary defense in the nose is the combination of the mucus holding on to the pollutants and the cilia sweeping it out, which goes on continuously without our awareness. The back up is the scrubbing, sneezing, and runny nose that so many find bothersome and that our pharmaceutical industry wrong-headedly focuses on turning off.

Consider that the most common triggers for asthma are actually allergens that look to the immune system like life threatening toxins (as in the case of cholera), or infectious agents like bacteria or viruses. Margie Profet, an evolutionary biologist, has shown how allergens share many characteristics with serious toxins and concludes that the response they trigger is a defense with a survival value. Paying attention to these toxins is what has led to one of the more common explanations of allergy yet—the hygiene hypothesis.

THE HYGIENE HYPOTHESIS

Several years ago researchers looking at allergies in European military recruits found that the problem was significantly less in recruits from rural farms where the barn and animals are adjacent to the house. These and other researchers pursuing this idea concluded that the significant exposure of serious toxins to the developing child at the right time helps their immune system to develop in a healthier way. The idea is known as the hygiene hypothesis and it is rapidly becoming accepted as a reason for allergies. It explains why we cannot survive well in a super sterile environment. The recognition of what is a serious toxin by our immune systems can be especially problematic when we live in a clean environment and have not been exposed to the normal bacteria, pollens and molds that are more common in less clean households and farming environments. A naive immune system that has not been exposed to a variety of toxins is more likely to consider allergens or irritants of lesser significance to be real dangers. This association has become apparent in many studies over the last few decades, and the benefits of less allergies include, of course, less asthma.

If a naive immune system, which has not been earlier exposed to these toxins and is therefore confused about the nature of the allergens/toxins it senses, is unable to get rid of them by washing then at least the nasal-bronchial reflex allows it to protect the lungs from what it considers a real danger. And that, I believe, is what happens with asthma. And that is why washing the nose is such an effective means of preventing asthma. It addresses the source of the problem.

The chemical that triggers the closing of the airway is histamine; the same histamine that causes the runny nose, that is the bad guy in allergies, and that all cold-pills (antihistamines) try to block. We will talk more about nasal defenses in the next chapter, but histamine is the trigger for the backup defense—and the defense is both washing and the shutting down of the airway to protect the lungs that we have turned into an illness that is called asthma. Obviously, no one questions the need for a good doctor during an acute episode. Yet to believe turning that defense off permanently or semipermanently will cure the patient is also wrong thinking.

There are two ways one can think about these defenses. On the one hand there are those believing that we were created by God the way we are. On the other hand are those who believe that we are the product of natural selection. Either way you look at it, however, these defenses are the best that are available; either God created them or they are expressed in us because of their success. To treat them appropriately we need to honor and support them, even when they are bothersome—and certainly not turn them off.

I attended a conference entitled Rethinking the Pathogenesis of Asthma some years ago in Santa Fe, New Mexico, where I presented some of these ideas. One of the speakers was Stephen Holgate, a recognized authority on the origins of asthma. He pointed out in his presentation that we have gone for thirty years with no new treatment for asthma, that it is caused by injury to the airway, and that what we need is a way to protect the airway from this injury. That, I told him, is what happens when you keep your nose clean. But this concept requires that we think differently about asthma and that is hard to get across, especially to the professionals who make their living off treating this disease.

But we are making some progress. The hygiene hypothesis is increasingly accepted because the evidence is so pervasive, but there is much foot dragging. Asthma is a condition that is hard to explain in the traditional view where one deals only with airway inflammation and constriction, without asking why. Medical researchers are most happy with simple causes that they can address easily with drugs. When we start talking about complex causes they get uneasy. The same kind of thing happened when Hans Selye started looking at how stress contributed to so many health problems; he was criticized for studying the impact of soil, or what some critics derisively simply termed 'dirt', on our health.

Unfortunately we live in a complex world and we are complex creatures, and we have to accept too that many of our illnesses are complex. Medical schools are stuck in the analytical model where the body is seen as a complicated machine—complicated but still capable of being analyzed. Such systems are easy to analyze because you can just connect the dots. But the dots in complex systems are networked and the number of interrelationships rapidly becomes unmanageable. Adaptive systems, like living agents are even more complex because they can adapt and create novelty. Adaptation is not a part of the analytical and mechanical way that doctors are taught and how they continue to see the body. Once the concept of adaptation is seen and accepted then the role of nasal defenses also becomes clear and the whole system of seeing the body as a complicated machine breaks down. That change in viewpoint is something the priesthood of medicine will resist to the end. In the peer review process, articles submitted to medical journals are selected or rejected by editors who work to maintain the dominant viewpoint, so the only journal that accepted two of my articles for publication that raised this question was the non-peer reviewed journal *Medical Hypotheses*. Not only are these editors persuaded by the dominant view, but also were they to publish something that decreased the profits of the pharmaceutical industry it would hurt their advertizing revenue, which is likely why *Medical Hypotheses* is on the brink of folding.

My point is that regularly washing the nose reduces exposure and allows the body to both learn about and better deal with these threats, both from allergens and infectious agents, without the challenge being too great.

When children are exposed to toxins such as these their immune systems have little trouble recognizing the bad guys; their immune systems become educated and they learn that ragweed or cedar are not really as bad as the other toxins. In the future we may possibly have easy and safe ways to expose our children to these toxins that will help avoid asthma and allergy problems. In the meantime we need to honor what our immune system is trying to do.

After the success we saw with Traci and her asthma I began using the spray more often with asthma patients; an early opportunity came when an 11-year old boy, with no prior history of asthma, came to my office wheezing with a peak flow of 150. Again, peak flow measures how much air a person can force out and gives a rough idea of the openness of the airway. A peak flow reading of 150 isn't very good, but it improved with an albuterol breathing treatment, so I gave him a prescription for an inhaler and a bottle of the spray and told him to clean his nose regularly for a few days. He did not get the albuterol inhaler, but he took the spray to the school nurse and every class break he would spray his nose. His peak flow over the next three days went from the 150 to 250, to 350, and to 450, which was normal for his size.

The stand-up comedian Chris Rock has a routine where he argues that doctors will never find a cure for AIDS as long as they make money off of treating it. A profit shifts the focus from prevention to making the symptoms livable. It's the same with asthma; the focus is on making the symptoms livable so few see the role of a clean nose in preventing the problem.

Researchers are getting around to looking at the question of how asthma is triggered, but it is slow going. The "one airway hypothesis" is based on the well-demonstrated fact that nasal irritants trigger a neurological response that results in bronchospasm. People studying asthma have some difficulty with the concept that the major triggers for asthma are in the nose, but this is what my patients tell me and they are not any different from all of the others suffering from asthma. The major triggers are allergies, sinus conditions and viral upper respiratory infections—all problems that begin in the nose.

When the nasal immune system identifies one of these irritants that it cannot wash out, even though it tries (as any person with allergic rhinitis can readily attest), it must focus on limiting the damage. If it cannot wash it out at least it can prevent it from getting into the deeper parts of the body where it may cause more serious problems. It does this by using the nasal-bronchial reflex to close down the airway—by damming up what it considers a polluted stream. Reflexes, as pointed out earlier, are always defenses that protect us, and the nasal-bronchial reflex that protects our lungs from perceived pollutants in the upper airway is a defense—asthma is a defense. We have been looking at the wrong aspects of asthma for the last 50 years. That's not very flattering to all of our researchers who are not attracted to this idea. But I can't explain the benefits I see any other way.

Just the other day I got some more confirmation for this idea. One of those letters that doctors get from the drug companies telling of another warning about their drug. This time the drug was salmeterol, marketed as Serevent and Advair. This drug is used as a long acting bronchodilator. It is not for use in acute episodes because it doesn't work fast enough. A study the drug company had done showed that over 28 weeks asthmatics who received salmeterol in addition to their other asthma medications died more frequently than if they received a placebo. The number was not great, 13 out of 13,174 versus 4 out of 13,179, but that is the kind of problems we see when we block a defense. The trend was even greater for African-American patients.

For patients with asthma, however, the nasal connection is often intuitive. I am not sure if I am not promoting some of this, but many of my asthma patients with whom I have spoken describe the sensation of an asthma attack as their body's response to triggers sensed in the nose.

THE PRIMARY DEFENSE—THE SWEEPING

If we could look with a microscope inside of an ideal nose we would see all of the pollutants and infecting agents stuck in mucus that coats and protects our airway, and the mucus would be moving slowly toward the back of the nose. Ideally it takes about 15 minutes for the mucus to move from the front of the nose to the back of the throat where we swallow it; then the acid and digestive enzymes in our stomach recycle all of the proteins in the mucus and destroy the pollutants. The mucus is secreted by special cells scattered among those lining our airway and swept by microscopic hairs called cilia that extend into the airway from the other cells in the airway; they normally wave about ten times every second. Between these ciliated and mucus secreting cells and the mucus layer is the airway surface fluid that provides some space so the cilia can sweep effectively, a liquid bed for the mucus to float on so it can be easily swept out, and some fluid for the mucus. Mucus is secreted in a concentrated form and rapidly absorbs large amounts of water. The airway surface fluid is also the home of several protein substances, called *defensins*, which help trap and kill foreign bacteria. These three elements, the mucus that does the trapping, the cilia that sweep it out, and the airway surface fluid that enables both to work effectively, make up what is called the mucociliary elevator—the primary defense for

Figure 3

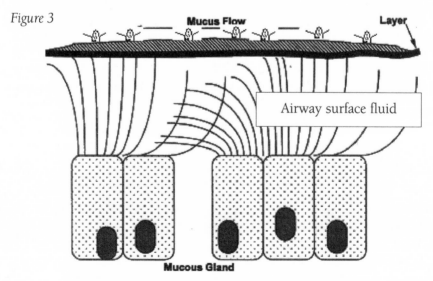

cleaning the airway. It cleans the upper airway by sweeping to the back of the nose and it sweeps the major parts of the airways in the lungs by sweeping upward; it even sweeps the Eustachian canals. In all areas it moves the mucus to the back of the throat where we swallow it. It works 24 hours a day and 7 days a week; it is a very effective cleaning mechanism when it is working properly. Figure 3 is a diagrammatic representation of this process with an optimal space for the airway surface fluid.

There are also several factors we have already mentioned that hurt it.

Smoking hurts the cilia so they don't work properly as well as loading the airway with lots of toxic chemicals. The cilia become disorganized and don't beat effectively and the airway soon shows indication of irritation and inflammation, notes M.A. Elliott and co-researchers in an article in the April 2007 issue of the *American Journal of Respiratory Cell and Molecular Biology*. For children this is even worse. We don't know which of these factors, the smoke or the toxins, is so damaging to the airway of smaller children, but the message is clear that we should not smoke around them.

Even clearer is the reason for the effect of dryness on your nasal defenses. Figure 4 is a representation of this cleaning process when it is handicapped: the mucus is dry and does not hold on effectively to the bacteria or other pollutants nor is it able to be moved out as easily; the cilia are disorganized, and the airway surface fluid is compromised and deficient.

Figure 4

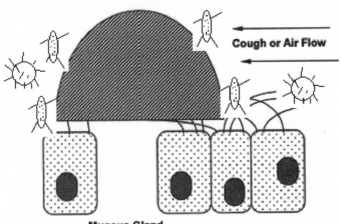

Cough or Air Flow

Mucous Gland

Mucus secreted in the nose rapidly absorbs water to increase its volume by several hundred times, and again, the wetter it is the better it works. It can get this water either from the airway surface fluid or from the moisture in the air, but if it is taken from the airway surface fluid, even though the volume of that fluid is replaced rapidly from the surrounding tissues, the cleaning mechanism is compromised. This underscores the importance of drinking enough water as well as trying to maintain a healthy humidity in the environment for the proper working of this cleaning action.

THE SCRUBBING—THE HISTAMINE RESPONSE

Just as some spills on the kitchen floor require more than a broom there are times when the mucociliary clearance is not up to the job of cleaning the nose. When pollutant sensing cells in the nose are triggered by foreign debris, toxins, or infecting agents they trigger the backup cleaning by releasing histamine. In the 1940s histamine was labeled a bad molecule; it triggered inflammation; inflammation was bad; therefore, histamine was the ENEMY. Most of our health care industry continues to think this way but some are coming around. Christer Svensson is a researcher from Sweden who used his electron microscope to look for any harmful effects in nasal tissue after a histamine challenge, as he reported in the January-February 1998 issue of the *American Journal of Rhinology*. Being unable to find any he concluded that histamine and the washing it triggers is actually a defense.

According to the American Academy of Allergy, Asthma, and Immunology, histamine does four things in the nose: first, it opens small blood vessels under the cells lining the nasal cavity so they leak; second, it increases the mucus; third, it's an irritant; and, finally fourth, it closes the airway.
- Opening the blood vessels does several things:
  - It provides the water for the washing; the fluid percolates up around the cells, bathing them in the process,
  - It replenishes and increases the airway surface fluid with its *defensins*,
  - It optimizes the water available for the mucus to be wet, sticky, and moveable, and thus helps it all get cleaned out faster and easier.
- Increasing the mucus is like adding a vacuum cleaner to the process. More mucus picks up more garbage.

- The local irritation increases the sneezing and as any mother can readily attest the socially unacceptable display of mucus coming from the nose is all too often brought on by a sneeze. But Mom, would you rather have the pollutants and the mucus holding them in your child's nose or out? This cleaning is a defense and the pollutants it is attempting to remove do cause problems in our bodies.
- The fourth effect of histamine is closing down the airway to protect the more vulnerable lungs.

Cough and cold pills shut down this back-up cleaning. These pills are made up of decongestants, which close down the opening of the blood vessels and turn off the water, and antihistamines which block the effects of histamine and turn off the whole process. And when one goes to the doctor with severe symptoms they are commonly given a shot or a prescription for steroids which turns off the immune system so it doesn't care if the nose is polluted. Honoring and supporting these defenses is a much better choice than using what is available from the wonders of modern medicine.

Our immune system is strongest in these openings to the body; it is there to recognize, identify, and build defenses against invaders. At the same time it operates throughout our body seeking out aberrant cells like those that turn into cancer. It needs to be optimal and we should think twice before taking drugs that handicap it or turn it off.

THE ASTHMA CONNECTION

The fourth effect of histamine, closing down the airway, needs further explanation. Closing the airway is a reasonable thing to do when one considers that the defenses in the lung are far less robust than those in the upper airway, and that should the pollutants get into the lungs they could wreak havoc there. But at the same time we do need to breathe. This is a case where the immune system can kill us, and we have made it into an illness we call asthma, but few see it as a defense that may be trying to protect us. Allergens are the most common trigger for asthma and many allergens look very similar to potent toxins. Margie Profit, the evolutionary biologist whom I mentioned, elaborated on this idea in an article, "The function of allergy: immunological defense against toxins," in the March 1991 *Quarterly Review of Biology*.

Of course no one calls it a defense or makes that connection; and they will not as long as the focus remains on how to deal with the symptoms instead of looking at the underlying cause. Asthma is triggered by agents outside the body. It's a disease condition characterized by airway inflammation and constriction mediated by an errant immune system that we can easily block with drugs. Few recognize or acknowledge that it is a part of our nasal defenses. It may be a defense that kills, but it is still a defense and defenses need to be honored; and honoring them does make them less aggressive.

These three elements make up the primary defense we have for cleaning our airway. It cleans the upper airway by sweeping to the back of the nose and it sweeps the major parts of the airways in the lungs by sweeping upward; as mentioned, it even sweeps the Eustachian canals. This defense needs to be supported, just as we support the defense of our favorite football team.

CHAPTER FIVE

Moisturizing with Xylitol

Jerry was off presenting at an educational conference the last time she had an episode of gastroenteritis. The other teachers with her were happy to get another room. They thought she was a bit quirky when she shut herself up with crackers and Pedialyte without the benefit of medical attention, but she was better the following day and they trusted her to drive them home. Our grandchildren have been around long enough to pick up and accept a few of these quirks. Now when they get feeling a bit congested or like they may be coming down with something they will ask for oral rehydration and they all have and use their own bottles of the nasal spray. The key here is helping defenses. Simple.

As for me, I could always tell that I was going to be busy with kids and upper respiratory infections soon after a West Texas cold spell. Like Jerry and the connection she saw between ear infections and special education, you know something connects these but you are not sure what it is. We all recognize that wintertime is the time for colds and flu, but hardly anyone asks why; those that do concentrate again on the bugs. Viruses can survive longer in cold air so this is proposed as the reason why they don't have a flu season in the tropics.

Everyone seems to have their own favorite treatment designed to thwart the wintertime bugs, but without understanding the why behind the problem they are more than likely anecdotal treatments that we associate with a particular success that was just as likely luck. Few look at how the weather affects our defenses. I believe that the underlying connection has to do with humidity and the nasal defenses it supports when it is in the optimal range.

Several years ago, to illustrate, we visited some of the smaller towns in Alaska and talked with the people who were trying to cope with all of the ear infections in the native population. These people have the highest incidence of ear infections in the country, and quite possibly in the whole world. Again, ear infections are the classic upper respiratory infection for children; bacteria climb down their Eustachian canals into the middle ear, just as they climb up into the sinuses in older people, but in both they begin their journey from their homes in the back of the nose.

The people we talked with were mostly audiologists and their helpers who went out into the native communities and talked with the people. One of the stories they heard repeatedly from the elders in these villages was that their people did not have ear infections before they were 'civilized.' When we asked the doctors about this story they said that the ear infections were there, but they were just not recognized. I am not sure about that; the natural history of an untreated ear infection is a painful ear that gets better immediately when the ear drum ruptures and the puss from the middle ear drains out. That's a pretty easy process to recognize so we didn't think that a doctor was needed to make the diagnosis; we believed the elders. Furthermore the people of Kotzebue's sister city of Provideniya, across the Bering Straits in Siberia, while they shared the same genetic base that included this disposition for ear infections, had neither the benefits of civilization nor a problem with ear infections at the time we were there.

In all fairness to the doctors, they are moved in and out of these frontier 'hardship' areas on a regular basis; they, unlike the technicians that we talked to, have little time to listen to the elders.

'Civilized' meant that they were taken from their native habitat and given prefab houses in which to live. While this new environment was far more comfortable, and no one seriously considers going back, it also significantly altered the context to which their bodies had adapted. Elders from other native groups, from the aborigines of Australia and New Zealand to the Native Americans of New Mexico, tell the same story: taking people from their native habitat makes them less healthy; and mostly the poor health is centered in the respiratory system. What's going on here?

Besides filtering and cleaning the air that we breathe the nose also has to warm it and humidify it. It normally does this so well that the air entering the lungs is almost always body temperature and 100 percent humid, even in a variety of environments. In cold environments this is a challenge that requires a great increase in blood flow to the nose and an almost constant flow of small amounts of histamine to help open the taps for fluid to get into the airway surface fluid, which plays the dominant role in providing the moisture to accomplish this task. Similar challenges face almost anyone living out of doors in a temperate environment. But it is a challenge that we have adapted to over thousands of years. It is far less of a challenge to someone who lives in the tropics where it is generally both warmer and more humid.

Most of the fluid needed for this warming and humidification comes from what we drink and the part of that that gets into the airway surface fluid, but there is some help from the environment. Some time ago some people looked at the effect of humidity on our illnesses and Figure 5 shows what they found:

Figure 5

Humidity and Nasal Problems

Effect of Humidity on Common Nasal Irritants

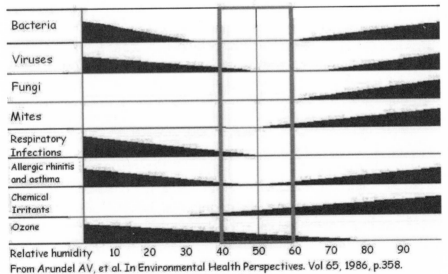

From Arundel AV, et al. In Environmental Health Perspectives. Vol 65, 1986, p.358.

This study together with what we have learned about how our airway defenses work is why we think humidity is a more defining reason for why we have a flu season. Specifically the airway surface fluid plays a critical part in helping the cilia and mucus to work best and it interacts with the air we breathe: it is replenished in moist air and reduced in dry air. In the tropics, where the humidity is most often in the healthy 40-60 percent range, the nose works better. In the temperate zones the humidity fluctuates more outside, but inside, when the central heating/cooling is on, the humidity is generally in the 20-30 percent range and the airway surface fluid has to make up the difference; if the person is not adequately hydrated the cleaning defense is handicapped. Notice in the chart that while high humidity is associated with more viruses and bacteria it is only when the air is dry that upper respiratory infections are increased; if there is enough moisture the nose can more easily wash the infecting agents out.

The process for most of us as we moved indoors and into our more efficient centrally heated and air conditioned environments has been slow enough that we did not notice this change in respiratory problems, while the natives, where the move was abrupt, did. People in the tropics live mostly with the windows, if there are any, open, and the humidity is usually in a healthy range. People living in the temperate zones have lower temperatures and must create their own ways to moderate their environment to make it comfortable. Until the advent of central heating they generally lit a fire somewhere to warm up. While the heat lowered the humidity there was always enough air coming in from outside, to compensate for the air that went up the chimney, that provided some moisture. When we moved to central heating we could increase the efficiency of the heating by closing off these drafts, but the humidity suffered. In a well insulated home with the central heating on we have a hard time getting the humidity above 30 percent.

For all of us living in the temperate zones the move indoors is recent in comparison to how long we have been around; and the move to central heating and cooling is less than a century old. It takes thousands of years for our bodies to adapt to physical changes in our environments and we have not had long enough for our noses to adapt to our drier, but more comfortable and artificial environments; and we have increased our insulation and isolation from outdoors and the efficiency of our heating and cooling systems only within the past 50 years.

Suffice it to say here that we need to take other actions to support the defenses we have handicapped in this process. As the risk factors associated with low humidity imply, until our bodies find a way to adapt to these changes we need to find a way to counter the harmful effects; we need to find a way to support these handicapped defenses. If we don't we will continue having our cold and flu season, more URIs, and no relief in our battle with allergens and asthma.

Water, after air, is the most critical element for a properly functioning body and most of us need to make a conscious effort to drink more. It's also the most critical element in the mucociliary elevator. Insufficient water means that the body doesn't have enough to properly fill the airway surface fluid, and the airway surface fluid doesn't have enough to hydrate the secreted mucus, and dry mucus is not as effective in both holding garbage and carrying it out. Drinking water and to a lesser extent humidity can provide water to the airway surface fluid. The importance of drinking enough water is a foundation of maintaining health. Water is the body's oil; just as oil is a necessary part of all machines the body needs water; but few of us drink the recommended three to four quarts a day. And we are fortunate if we are able to have more than 30 percent humidity in our insulated and centrally heated homes. Adding to the humidity with a humidifier, vaporizer, or even a pot of water on the stove is energy intensive, and in my own case led to many burned out pots. Using a humidifier requires regular cleaning to prevent molds.

Moving to the tropics where the humidity is higher offers little help today because we take our air conditioners with us, and cooling the air in this way also dries it. Swamp coolers work by putting water into the air and are healthier in dry environments, but they don't work well in most of the country, or most of the tropics, where summer air is both hot and wet.

Stopping smoking is always a wise thing to do, especially of you are bothered by a respiratory problem or have children around. If you must smoke then take a hint from the natives. Among indigenous people smoking was practiced wherever tobacco was available, and it was a sacred practice. Smoking made the breath, the life giving vital force, visible. Generally it was a shared practice, much like communion in Christian churches. So if you must smoke (and I really wish you wouldn't) make it sacred: roll your own; share your cigarette with someone you care for. You will smoke less and enjoy it more; and it will be a mindful practice, as it should be, and not the mindless habit that it mostly is today. Turning sacred practices into mindless habits always seems to rob them of their significance—and the gods wind up biting you in the rear—and smoking is no exception. And if you must smoke make sure you compensate for handicapping your defense by regularly washing your nose as well as encouraging those around you to do the same.

A common alternative to a dry airway in the U.S. is to moisten it with small bottles of saline that make a mist for inhaling when you squeeze them. These sprays became popular around the same time the use of antihistamines was increasing and they do a reasonable job countering the dry nose these drugs caused. They even help reduce the incidence of infections. Researchers at Harvard have found people they call heavy polluters who breathe out large amounts of viruses and bacteria. The simple inhalation of vaporized saline eliminates this pollution within minutes, likely by making the mucus stickier for a few minutes.

If saline is effective at reducing the bacteria we breathe out one would think that it should also reduce respiratory infections, and it does; but not by much. My own experience is characteristic. I began using a nasal saline spray soon after I began practice to deal with the occupational hazard of respiratory infections. They didn't eliminate the problem, but they did cut it by about a third—maybe half. Because of this benefit I have recommended the use of these sprays often and aggressively in children with ear infections, but they didn't seem to help at all in these problems. Something else was needed.

We talked earlier about the Native Americans in Alaska and the problem they have with ear infections since they were civilized. Several years ago a group of researchers at Johns Hopkins were looking at the effect of cold on the nose. Cold air cannot hold as much moisture as warmer air so it tends to dry the airway surface fluid and make what is left more concentrated. In order to mimic this condition they got volunteers to put 5 mls (about a teaspoon) of a concentrated solution of mannitol (a close form of the sugar mannose that is common in the body) into their nose and hold it there for a few seconds before letting it drain back out. When they examined what came out they found that it had more volume—the mannitol had worked osmotically to pull more fluid into the nose—and that there was a small amount of histamine present. The presence of histamine was enough to stop this line of research because it was considered then a cause of inflammation. When one stops to realize, however, that histamine is the trigger for nasal washing and that it, as Dr. Svensson pointed out, is a critical part of this defense, its presence here as a response to this challenge, is perfectly understandable. The task of hydrating and warming air when one lives in a very cold environment requires the increased blood flow that histamine triggers. Consider also that the concentrated mannitol pulls fluid into the nose from the cells in a manner that is functionally identical to the bathing of the cells done by histamine, and one realizes that osmotic agents such as this may be very useful in washing the airway. The fluid they stimulate goes into the airway surface fluid where it can be used to adequately hydrate the newly secreted mucus. This may be helpful as the something else that is more effective than just saline.

The need for something else became critical when Heather began having ear infections. After her fourth infection, when her doctor opened the subject of tubes, Jerry's thirty-year old memories returned with a vengeance. During the intervening years she had become a psychotherapist with an appreciation of reality therapy, which she used on me: "WHAT YOU ARE DOING ISN'T WORKING," she said, "DO SOMETHING ELSE,"—and she meant it. While I wasn't our granddaughter's doctor her parents had tried my suggestion of frequent saline spraying, but it did not help in her case either, even though the idea is right; moistening the airway should help it clean itself more effectively. But it didn't prevent her infections; something else was needed. That was when the article from the *British Medical Journal* about the Finnish researchers reducing the incidence of ear infections by having children regularly chew gum sweetened with xylitol caught my attention.

Xylitol is an interesting substance. First of all it is not a drug; it is a natural plant sugar. Plants use xylose like animals use glucose. Xylitol is white and crystalline. It looks and tastes like sugar and has been used as a sugar substitute for many years. It has been evaluated by the Food and Drug Administration as a food, specifically a sugar substitute, and placed in the category they call GRAS—generally recognized as safe. Similar agencies around the world accept this classification.

It is especially useful for diabetics with a sweet tooth because it is metabolized differently than glucose and doesn't need insulin; and it doesn't raise glucose levels when it is eaten. Finland is one of the places where xylitol is used more because they can make it from their birch trees and don't have to import sugar. One of the benefits the Finns found early on was xylitol's effect on preventing tooth decay, which will be the subject of a later chapter.

The information in this study looking at children, gum and ear infections was interesting, but it didn't really help much because Heather was only 9 months old and not quite up to chewing gum. Again the authors pointed out that the xylitol worked on the bacteria, and as we point out those bacteria are in the back of the nose, so it made sense to put it there. We gave our son a bottle of spray with xylitol my hospital pharmacy had mixed up for me and suggested that they spray Heather's nose at every diaper change. Her ear infections went away. So did those of the children in my 'Ears and Fears Study' discussed earlier in the introduction.

I was not able to follow up on the one child who had three ear problems during the period I watched them. I could not determine, for example, if those administering the spray were doing it right or not, nor get samples from his middle ear for finding out what kind of bacteria were present. There are certainly bacteria that don't respond to xylitol, but it seems that the vast majority of the ones causing problems do.

XYLITOL AND BACTERIAL ADHERENCE

I already mentioned that I called Dr. Matti Uhari, the lead researcher in the chewing gum/ear infection study, after I found out how putting xylitol in the nose was so much more effective in preventing ear infections than its oral use. Besides encouraging me to reproduce his studies, he told me about a study his group had done that was awaiting publication. In it they showed why xylitol was so effective nasally.

This study was done in the laboratory and not in people. They took cells from the nose and helped them to grow on artificial membranes. These are the cells that bacteria learn to hold on to when they establish a home in the back of the nose. Then they selected bacteria that cause the most infections when they hold on to these cells and picked strains of these bacteria that were the most virulent. They divided both the cells and the bacteria into two groups and put a little bit of xylitol in one part of each. Then they put them all together in four different sets: one with no xylitol in either cell or bacteria, one with xylitol in both, and one each with xylitol in either the cell or the bacteria. They let them alone for a while to bond, then washed them and counted the number of bacteria still holding on to each cell. Figure 6 shows their results. It is clear that xylitol has an effect on the adherence of these major nasal pathogens, but mostly on the major pathogen, *Streptococcus Pneumoniae*, where the combination of xylitol on both bacteria and cells reduced the ability of these bacteria to hold on by 68 percent.

Figure 6

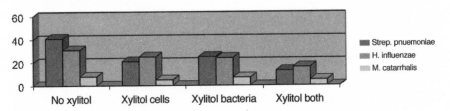

Kontiokari T, Uhari M, Koskela M. "Antiadhesive effects of xylitol on otopathogenic bacteria," *J Antimicrob Chemother.* 1998 May;41(5):563-5.

The authors pointed out again, as they had in the ear infection study, that this interference is most likely due to competition at the binding sites. This competition requires relatively large amounts of the competing sugar that were readily available in the lab, but certainly not in the nose when the xylitol was put in the mouth. I don't know why they didn't consider putting it in the nose; it seemed reasonable.

What bacteria hold on with are numerous molecular-sized hands called lectins that are shaped specifically for their particular receptors. Receptors are what they hold on to. These receptors are almost always specific sugar complexes on the surfaces of our cells. Nathan Sharon, one of the earliest researchers to look at this adherence mechanism, said the lectins have a sweet tooth.

Sharon looked, for example, at the way *E. coli* hold on in the bladder. These are the bacteria that cause most urinary tract infections and he found that they hold on to mannose molecules, which are plentiful on the cell surfaces in the genital tract and the bladder. He also suggested that putting mannose in this environment would compete at these binding sites and fill up the bacterial lectins so that they could not hold on to the bladder. It's a well known process called competitive inhibition, and it works. But mannose is one of the more common sugars found in the body; it is a natural substance that cannot be patented so again: no patent—no profit; no profit—no research; no research—no drug, and no one knows.

Fortunately there is a sugar that works about a tenth as well as mannose that is available and well known for this purpose, because grandmother's advice to her daughters to drink cranberry juice to prevent urinary infections most likely works on this basis. There is hardly any mannose in cranberry juice but there is lots of fructose, and fructose has been shown to compete at *E. coli* binding sites, but not as well as the mannose does.

Drinking cranberry juice is not a very effective way to get it into the bladder where it can act directly on these bacteria, but this may not even be necessary. Most urinary tract infections in women begin from bacteria in their own GI tracts. The bacteria get into the bladder because of poor hygiene, like wiping the wrong way, or they can even migrate in bath water. If the GI tract is their reservoir then addressing the problem there should be just as effective; and research shows that it is. As the person eats the fructose, or drinks the cranberry juice, the infection causing bacteria latch on to this sugar and can't then hold on in the bowel. They are gradually replaced by strains of bacteria that don't hold on to these sugar complexes and can't cause urinary tract infections.

There is also one study that shows long-term benefits. Long-term benefits mean that the benefits continue after the treatment ends. In the case of illnesses caused by bacteria the continued benefits mean that either the bacteria are not there anymore, or they have changed in their nature to not cause the problem any longer. Taking an appropriate antibiotic for an infection confers a long-term benefit because the infecting bacteria are gone, but it has the down side of stimulating antibiotic resistance and killing off friendly bacteria as well as the ones causing the infection. There is no down side to using sugars to negotiate with bacteria. We will see more long-term benefits when we talk about tooth decay.

The same group in Finland that did the xylitol ear infection study did a study showing long-term benefits in treating urinary infections, but the long-term part was an accident. They looked at women who had chronic urinary infections; their infections kept coming back despite their regular use of antibiotics. The study used a combination of lingonberry and cranberry extracts and was to last a year; and it did, despite the fact that the producer of the extract went out of business half way through the study. That was the accident that made this study so interesting; these women were only treated for six months, while they could get the extract, but they were watched for a year—long enough to show that they received a long-term benefit. Figure 7 is our adaptation of their graphic results that shows this long-term benefit. If

Figure 7

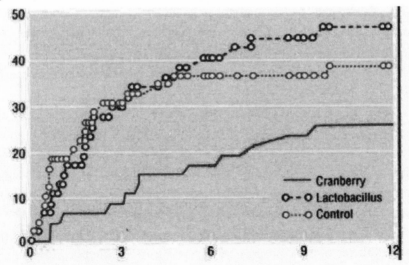

Kontiokari T, et al. Randomised trial of cranberry-lingonberry juice and Lactobacillus GG drink for the prevention of urinary tract infections in women, *BMJ* 2001 Jun 30;322(7302):1571-76.

cranberry juice works to acidify the urine or to kill the bacteria, both of which have been claimed and looked at by the cranberry juice industry, then these women should have begun getting infected again after they ran out of the extract, but they didn't. They received a long-term benefit that again comes either from the bacteria not being there any more, or their having become domesticated so they don't attack us; those are the only options open to us to explain long-term benefits when dealing with infections or other conditions caused by bacteria.

We will look again at long-term benefits when we talk about xylitol and tooth decay, and again when we talk about warfare with bacteria. It is an important topic that is not understood in our current model where the focus is on destroying our enemies. It helps us to understand a better way of dealing with our pathogens—and xylitol plays a large part.

The study that Matti Uhari told me about was not the first to show xylitol able to block bacterial adherence. Earlier studies by researchers in the Netherlands had shown it to block the adherence of *Clostridium difficile*, bacteria that often cause problems in the GI tract after we kill off the friendly bacteria with antibiotics. And later studies by the Japanese have shown it to block the adherence of several strains of Staphylococci, even multi-resistant *Staphylococcus aureus*. Add this ability of xylitol to inhibit bacterial adherence to that already described about its ability to block biofilm formation and adherence and you can get a sense of what xylitol can do to help our defenses. It is like soap for the nose; and not only does it unhook the bacteria and harmful biofilm, but it brings in more water by its osmotic effects to more effectively wash them all out.

This osmotic effect turned out to be the focus of a group at Iowa that began looking at using xylitol to treat children with cystic fibrosis shortly after the Finns demonstrated its adherence blocking ability. They looked a bit further at what xylitol does in the airway and found that it acts locally as an osmotic agent that pulls water into the airway. This is good for most children with cystic fibrosis because their mucus is dry and doesn't work very well so they get upper and lower respiratory infections all of the time and most of these children die early because of them. They applied for and were granted a patent for aerosolized xylitol, where it is delivered to the lower airway by breathing with a nebulizer. This route is more amenable to profitable patenting because nebulizers are already controlled as medical devices.

This group looked specifically at the effect of xylitol on the airway surface fluid. They found that more fluid lowers the salt concentration and helps the antibiotic *defensins* there to work more effectively. It also provides water for more optimally wetting the mucus and more volume so that the cilia can move a bit more effectively.

Second, they found that the xylitol was not absorbed, that it acts locally; which adds much to its safety profile, and to our presentation to the FDA about its equivalence to plums. If it is not absorbed then it just gets moved to the back of the throat with all of the mucus and swallowed.

Third, they found that when a solution of xylitol was regularly sprayed into the noses of a group of volunteers it substantially decreased the number of bacteria there; after four days of regular use the reduction in bacteria was six times greater in those sprayed with xylitol than sprayed using only saline. This finding does much to support and explain my own experience on saline not working well.

Fourth, they found that xylitol did not aid the growth of a wide variety of harmful bacteria. Most of the bacteria that infect animals eat six carbon sugars, the basic sugars for animals. Xylose is a five carbon sugar. It is plant sugar, and while there are wide varieties of bacteria that infect plants and can eat five carbon sugars, they are not usually the ones that infect animals.

Later studies done by this group on the airway surface fluid in the bronchi show that xylitol stays around for about four hours. This supports and explains our finding that frequent use is more helpful.

In accordance with FDA standards and laws the company licensing and manufacturing this product makes no drug claims; all it does is clean your nose. After four years on the market it was voted BEST NEW NATURAL MEDICINE by America's health food stores. The company manufacturing and distributing this spray wishes that the award would have been BEST NEW NATURAL NASAL SOAP, which would have avoided some contacts with the FDA. The best compliment, however, is that the spray has been copied. The copies, however, are not as effective. On the recommendation of Heather's father we had patented the use of xylitol nasally, so while those copying the spray could say on the label "contains xylitol" the amounts were less than those in our patent and not effective. If you are confronted with a choice read the ingredients list. Xylitol should be the first listed after water if it is going to be effective. The same warning, or advice, holds for the gum containing xylitol. Here xylitol should be the first ingredient if you are going to get its full benefit at preventing tooth decay.

CHAPTER SIX

War with Bacteria

One way to look at xylitol is as the horse whisperer of the bacterial and viral world. Xylitol tames the wild beasts feeding in your nose. Warfare has always been a part of our lives in America. We were born of a Revolutionary War, preserved by a Civil War, and made safe by a series of wars against our enemies, beginning with the Indians and now with terrorists.

Our bodies are also periodically involved in warfare. Bacteria and viruses regularly invade us and could cause us to be seriously ill were it not for the immune system in each of us that deals with most of these agents before they can bother us. When we do get signs of an infection we generally rely on antibiotics to help us destroy the invading agents.

Our economy flourishes during wartime. National debt goes up to support the war economy, whether the war is cold or hot. In much the same way the pharmaceutical and health care industries benefit from our warfare with bacteria. But endless warfare is costly and many empires, like the ancient Greeks and Romans, collapsed in large part because of them; there is also a real link in humans between our illnesses and financial collapse.

Technology has played a large part in who wins our wars. Rifles won out over the bow and arrow, guided missiles over artillery; even the stirrup played a role by giving the mounted warrior more stability. The arms race is the attempt to maintain a position of strength with our enemy. But even when one side is clearly dominant there is always a way to fight back. One-sided overwhelming technical superiority breeds unconventional warfare as we have seen with guerrilla warfare and terrorism.

Our arms race with bacteria occurs when we use antibiotics to kill the infecting agent and the agent develops ways to get around them. The resistance they develop prompts us to develop the next generation of more potent antibiotics, and the cycle continues. As discussed earlier the race is even manifest in our immunizations; our immunization for pneumonia is directed at helping our immune systems recognize and kill the more problem causing strains of Streptococcus pneumoniae, and it is becoming less effective since it just opens the doors for other strains. A similar problem is present with our immunization to whooping cough where bacteria are showing resistance and infections increasing. On the other hand our immunizations for tetanus and diphtheria have been around for decades and are still as effective as they were when first developed; and there is no sign of resistant bacteria. The difference between these two types of immunization is that the long lasting group addresses not the bacteria but the toxins they elaborate, and the problematic immunizations trigger a response aimed at the bacteria themselves.

Bacteria, like all living agents, sense and adapt to their environments; and bacteria are the experts at this process. When challenged with antibiotics, or in any other way, bacteria increase their rate of mutation to find a way to cope with the threat. Again, not all of them do so, but enough that they are more often successful at finding a way around the challenge. When they are not directly challenged, as with the longer lasting immunizations that address only their toxins, there is no threat and the bacteria sense no need to respond. In this way, the long-lasting immunizations also work to domesticate the problematic bacteria.

Anything we can do to create this kind of contextual pressure on the bacteria that infect us is a step in the right direction. Isolation does this for all infectious diseases; screening windows does it for those carried by insects; condoms do it for sexually transmitted infections; and washing hands and noses does it for most other socially communicable diseases. We need to promote all of these measures.

Besides developing resistance these infecting agents may even fight back in different ways. David Satcher, when he was head of the CDC, pointed out that in a 21-year period in the midst of this war some 22 previously unknown agents or infectious diseases were discovered. Some of these are guerrilla fighters, like the bacteria that cause ulcers and the virus that causes AIDS, which remain camouflaged while they infect us. One is even a suicide bomber—the Ebola virus kills the host so rapidly that the virus doesn't have time to spread to another person.

We have turned bacteria into evil, the dark side, the terrorists against whom we must wage all out bomb warfare. Bombs being antibiotics. We also see bacteria and viruses as evil. We want them all dead. We sell antibacterial soap and bleach our countertops to kill germs that may be there. And they are there. Bacteria are everywhere. Ten percent of our own dry body weight is those bacteria that live with us, at least fifty percent of our DNA is straight from bacteria, and there are ten times more bacteria in our bodies than the larger cells of which we are made. They, like our macro enemies, are not necessarily evil. Bacteria are totally responsible for creating the balance that allowed life on this world and they are primarily responsible for the recycling that maintains that balance; and we have already discussed their role in our defenses by the barriers they provide and their help in our digestion and in making vitamins. Nor are they ignorant. By releasing chemicals in the process of quorum sensing that we talked about earlier bacteria are able to communicate with each other and act like a much larger organism. When left alone they make biofilm that is often as elaborate on a bacterial scale as the skyscrapers of New York. They also help each other by sharing genetic information, not only among their own type, but with any bacteria they come in contact with. Not having an interest in intellectual property rights this cooperation is one reason we are always playing catch-up in our arms race with them.

As a nation we recently fought a preventive war. When under pressure we always go back to our first principles. But as Hegel pointed out in his historical writings: Institutions are destroyed, in the end, by an excess of their first principles. The questions are, "Are we as a nation violent to excess, and is this one of our first principles that will end up destroying us?" The rest of the world seems to respond to the first overwhelmingly in the affirmative. The average American appears not to think so.

Sometimes we fight preventive wars with bacteria by taking antibiotics when we are at risk of being infected. Much of our antibiotics are used in the livestock industry for this reason, but also because antibiotics promote growth; and this use is largely unregulated. We are finding, however, that the benefit of reduced infections in humans and animals is not worth the cost of the bacterial resistance that comes from the increased exposure to the antibiotic. The most effective way to stop antibiotic resistance is to reduce our reliance on and use of antibiotics. This was actually demonstrated recently.

The Plexus Institute tries to find effective ways to deal with our real but complex problems. Working in cooperation with several hospitals and utilizing a program they call positive deviance they have addressed the issue of bacterial resistance, especially focusing on MRSA (methicillin resistant *Staphylococcus aureus*). At a recent nursing conference the director of the Plexus Institute, Curt Lindberg, described their results. Most of the measures developed using positive deviance are those that block bacterial transmission, like those along the lines proposed by Paul Ewald in his book, *The Evolution of Infectious Disease*, which we will get more into later. Lindberg related at this conference that the CDC, which had been monitoring the bacteria at these cooperating hospitals, reported that the *Staph. aureus* remaining after the positive deviance actually had lost some of their resistance. That is exactly what we should expect from such measures because the bacteria are adapting to their context and if there is no increase threat in that context they will adapt toward less resistance. Antibiotics kill bacteria; they are a threat—and they lead to resistance. Reducing antibiotics is the time-tested way to decrease resistance; and addressing and blocking their transmission is now shown to do this as well; and we argue that blocking adherence of the bacteria accomplishes the same thing. There are also other options for dealing with infectious diseases.

SENSIBLE AND COST EFFECTIVE, BUT NOT GLAMOROUS

Paul Ewald expresses the hope that we can "domesticate [bacteria] so that they can live with us in a less damaging way than they have throughout our history." We can do this, he argues, by addressing the areas that make it easy for the infecting agents to get from one person to another. We did this with cholera by public health measures that cleaned our water supplies, and we can do it for HIV with condoms and needle exchanges. In the case of cholera these barriers to spread actually change the outlaw agents to types that are less virulent, and Ewald claims the same trend is present with HIV/AIDS in Uganda and Japan where monogamy and condoms are openly and widely promoted. This is the kind of change that leads to the long-term benefits discussed earlier when bacteria change their nature. Epidemic cholera killed millions, but the cholera that has followed cleaning up water supplies is the El Tor strain where the mortality rate is almost negligible. More examples will be discussed in a later chapter on tooth decay.

This kind of isolation has never been tried with outlaw nations. Our best efforts have been in economic blockades and sanctions. The economic blockade of Cuba and the sanctions on Iraq destroyed much of the infrastructure of these countries, but not the regime. If anything these outside threats, just like in bacteria, tend to promote defensive adaptations that just increase hostility. If education and a middle class are necessary for the spread of democratic values the sanctions have probably done more harm than good. If we want these countries to shape up a policy more in line with what works with bacteria may be better: find a way to change their context so that they adapt in a friendlier way.

SIMPLE AND REASONABLE, BUT UNCONTROLLABLE AND INEXPENSIVE, SO NOT EVEN TRIED

Nathan Sharon and his colleagues have been arguing for at least twenty years that sugars can be effectively used to prevent infectious disease. Bacteria attach to specific sugar complexes on the cell surfaces in our bodies and if they can't attach to these sugars they are washed out and don't cause infection. Feeding the proper sugars to the bacteria fills up their hungry hands leaving them with no means of attaching; it decreases their adherence to the cells in our bodies. Regular use of such sugars also isolates the infectious agents in Ewald's sense, and selects for bacteria that cause less problems as we saw with E. coli and urinary infections. The sugars in cranberries select for bacteria that don't cause urinary tract infections. Xylitol decreases the adherence of problem causing bacteria in the nose, and selects for bacteria that cause less problems there. Bacteria that live in the nose without causing problems, cause sinus, ear, and bronchial infections when they move out of the nose and into these neighboring areas. Putting these sugars into the appropriate bacterial environment doesn't kill or threaten bacteria; it just fills up their hungry hands and gives them something to hold on to besides us. Sharon thinks that these sugars may be a part of the bacterial communication system; and what they seem to say to the bacteria is essentially 'shape up or ship out.' When they are used regularly that is what happens as the sugars compete at the binding sites so the bacteria can't hold on and are then easily washed out of our bodies.

The problem with these sugars is that they have to be used every day, even when there is no sign of infection; this message—to shape up or ship out— is best delivered regularly. Women drank cranberry extract every day for 6 months, but they had protection from urinary infections for a year. Our ancestor who first fed the wolf cooked meat had to feed them every day, for a long, long time, before the wolf became dog, and our best friend. Maybe we can do the same with bacteria. Ewald thinks it's possible and using sugars to negotiate makes it a whole lot easier.

These bacterial adaptations give us examples for how all animals adapt— including humans. If we change their environment in ways that attack the agent, pressure is applied for them to adapt defensively to cope with the threat—they become stronger and more determined enemies. If we change the environment in ways that are not threatening, they are more likely to adapt toward living with the host—toward domestication; Joseph Nye calls it 'soft power' and shows how it works, even in international relations.

I live in the Bible Belt in the middle of the Texas panhandle. In our community we take pride in our Christian heritage and that our nation is based on Christian principles. In searching for what it means to be a Christian I keep coming up with the "Sermon on the Mount" where Jesus says, "Love your enemies, bless them that curse you, do good to them that hate you, and pray for them which despitefully use you, and persecute you." This difficult task is, to me, the litmus test of a real Christian. Doing good to our enemies by feeding them worked in the Philippines, where guerrilla fighters were given jobs as they gave up their arms. But most of the time we tend to feed others with more armaments rather than addressing their basic needs as we perpetuate the use of hard power around the world.

Ever since Pasteur discovered the bacteria that cause anthrax and came up with the germ theory we have been at war with these microbes. Early on in this war we thought the enemy was only an aggressor that was trying to kill us. It wasn't until relatively recently that we realized how really dependent we are on the bacteria living in us and with us. They are a significant part of the primary defenses in all of those vulnerable open areas of our bodies where their friendly biofilm protects us from countless pathogens. This is especially true in the gastrointestinal and the female genital tract, but it holds for the nose and upper respiratory tract as well. And it has only been more recently yet that we began thinking about the effect of our antibiotics on these friendly bacteria. Few have heard about these concerns because the profits from antibiotics still weighs heavily on our 'conventional wisdom,' that part of our cultural mindset that James Galbraith says is there because there is a financial benefit somewhere. We do know now that killing off all of the bad bacteria is neither practical nor possible. We need these other options. Xylitol for washing your nose is one of the smartest options. Who would have thought that we would be making docile pets of these once predaceous bacterial strains?

Xylitol is like soap for the nose, and a soap that can be used regularly and easily. The frequent use of soap and water on the hands is accepted as the easiest and best way to stop the spread of communicable diseases. Easier, better, and more effective is washing your nose as often with a spray containing an adequate amount of xylitol. The bacteria and viruses don't get into our bodies through our hands but we introduce them ourselves when we rub our eyes or nose. Of course, we should wash our hands, but it also makes sense to wash the nose.

CHAPTER SEVEN

Viruses, Your Nose, and Coping With the Flu

I mentioned the conversation Jerry had with a second year medical student in Sweden about her favorite subject of ear infections and the educational problems that come from them. The medical student dismissed most of her concerns because, he claimed, viruses cause the majority of ear infections, so they don't require or benefit from antibiotic treatment. Some evidence for his position comes from the common finding that about 20 percent of the fluid from infected ears shows only a virus, most commonly a respiratory virus like the respiratory syncytial virus (RSV) that is a particular problem in infants and toddlers where those infected with it commonly develop asthma. It is also common for ear infections to follow a viral upper respiratory infection; some 20-50 percent of ear infections in clinical practice do so. On the other hand doctors looking at children with chronic ear infections took samples from the middle ear when these children had tubes placed in their eardrums to treat their chronic infections. All of the samples were positive by genetic testing for at least one bacterial pathogen and 92 percent of them had indication of biofilm in the middle ear. Again biofilms are the safe-houses that bacteria build and hide in to avoid discovery or antibiotics.

A discussion of the role of viruses and ear infections is important because these infections are the typical upper respiratory infection; but, unlike the medical student with whom Jerry spoke, I, on the other hand, would argue that viruses and bacteria seem to work together. If we can prevent the bacterial infections that commonly follow viral infections we will be ahead in the end. If we can prevent the viral infections we will be even further ahead. Keeping your nose clean can do both.

In order to do this we need to know a little about how these differing organisms get into the body as well as the defenses we all have to prevent this from happening.

We have already discussed how bacteria invade us. Mostly entering the body through its normal openings—the mouth, nose, and genitourinary tract—the bacteria must then find a place to hold on. Once they are established they begin multiplying. It is usually at this point that the immune system recognizes a problem and mounts a response. If the bacteria can avoid detection and continue growing they will soon get to the point when some of the bacteria begin building the biofilm that becomes their home and hideout.

It's different with viruses. They not only have to hold on, they have to get inside a cell in order to multiply. They use the genetic machinery in our own cells to reproduce and destroy the cell in the process. Understanding this process I have to wonder how the viruses that are supposed to cause 20 percent of ear infections get to the middle ear. The middle ear is not in the main channel of the respiratory tract, it's essentially up stream at the end of a branch of that tract we have named the Eustachian canal. It's a long way on a viral scale and these viruses don't often get into the bloodstream that would make movement throughout the body easier. The most reasonable answer to this transportation problem is the close association that viruses and bacteria have. When sampling middle ear fluid in children with ear infections the most common finding is *both* viruses and bacteria. Viruses open the doors for many bacteria to more easily infect us and it is just as likely that bacteria operate as taxicabs for viruses. A few years ago I read a book by Lewis Thomas, who could think out of the box enough to turn evolution on its head; he suggested that higher organisms, including humans, may just be technological developments of bacteria to enable them to get around better— bacteria may be taxicabs for viruses, but we may be taxicabs for the bacteria.

Different viruses attach to and enter different cells. Respiratory viruses enter cells lining the respiratory tract. Some viruses, like polio and the chicken pox virus that causes shingles pick on nerve cells. Others pick on different organs like the liver, or the brain. All of them, along with all other infecting organisms, appear to follow Paul Ewald's concept of evolving toward living with the host in a peaceful symbiotic relationship if they are sufficiently isolated or, in transportation parlance, if we handicap the taxis. He points out that even the virulent strains of HIV Japanese men pick up in Indonesia are tamed when they go back to Japan where condom use is much more prevalent and accepted. And again, the 1919 flu pandemic was likely as deadly as it was in part because the crowded conditions in the hospital tents allowed for the easy transmission of the virus to another host, which enabled it to mutate in a more virulent direction.

The direction of the medical community has been to encourage the use of drugs that fight the viruses; that avenue has been our traditional and relied upon means of dealing with all infectious diseases. But, as Ewald points out, that approach just perpetuates the war. A recent study in the *British Medical Journal* also raises some questions as to the benefits of using antiviral drugs on children with the flu. First of all the drugs shorten the flu symptoms by only a day where the illness usually lasts about a week. Secondly they don't relieve any of the usual bacterial infections that commonly follow the flu. They have little effect on post-infectious asthma (which often worsens) or the use of antibiotics, which usually involves an ever escalating cycle of medication. Finally, as others have pointed out, the drugs themselves are often the problem. The earliest of these new drugs oseltamivir (Tamiflu®) now comes with a warning mandated by the FDA that its use can be associated with serious psychological and neurological side effects: panic attacks, delusions, depression, loss of consciousness, and even suicide.

The version of the flu that poses a current problem around the world (swine flu or H1N1) is similar to that of 1919, which is a reason for so much concern. If it is as deadly as the earlier version we are in for trouble, but so far those having the current version have had relatively mild symptoms. We need to keep it that way. And we can do this by remembering what we have learned from our prior mistakes in putting sick people together and enabling the infecting agents to focus on getting more powerful. Blocking their ability to get around pushes infecting agents in the other direction:

• Washing hands often hampers transmission from person to person.

- Keeping hands away from face prevents the virus, if it does get to your hands, from getting into your body.
- Wash your nose every time you wash your hands. Carry your bottle of xylitol wash. If the virus does get into your nose from riding on particles in the air you want your nasal defenses optimal to prevent the virus from getting to the cells lining your airway. That's the job of the mucus and it is optimal if it is wettest, so drink plenty of fluids as well.
- Small particle masks can help prevent these particles from getting into your airway. Viruses are too small to be filtered out by the masks, but most viruses hitch rides on other particles, like bacteria, water droplets, or other 'taxis' to get around, and these are large enough to get stopped.
- If you get sick stay home! Isolation works! Don't enable the virus to adapt toward increased virulence by spreading it around.
- If you have other symptoms that may be defenses like fever or nasal congestion don't take drugs that block them. For a fever make yourself comfortable and drink plenty of fluids. For nasal congestion use the nasal spray with xylitol every 15 minutes for a few times until the nose is clear. For help in this you might consult your local biologist; most doctors haven't gotten around to seeing things this way yet.

NETI POTS FOR NASAL DEFENSES

One increasingly common way to help promote our nasal defenses is washing the nose with a neti pot. Our son is allergic to grass, but he persists in mowing his own lawn. After he is through, however, he needs to spend a few minutes with his neti pot.

For those of you not familiar with these devices they look like a traditional version of Aladdin's lamp. You put a saline solution in the top and pour it out through the spout into your nose. Bend over the sink, turn your head to the side, pour a little bit of water into the top most nostril, and it will drain out of the lower one. It's a neat and simple way to wash the nose that has been around for centuries. It has even been found to reduce the incidence of colds and upper respiratory problems in many clinical studies.

In May 2009, Dr. Mehmet Oz, in his appearances on *Oprah* after five years, spoke once more of the benefit of using a neti pot for nasal cleansing.

Dr. Oz, popularly known as "America's Doctor," has been a vocal proponent of the use of neti pots over the last few years. It is his focus on this ancient oriental practice that has brought the neti pot out of obscurity and made this ancient secret a popular mainstream phenomenon. "Whether called nasal irrigation, nasal lavage, neti-potting, or sinus irrigation," says Dr. Oz, "When you use it properly, it reduces dust and other contaminants in the nose, and it's a very effective way to clean the sinuses." Modern studies are showing that it's as effective as drugs for preventing sinus infections. Regular use of a neti pot is also hugely beneficial for people with nasal allergies and headaches, he said in an interview with *Healthy Living* magazine.

Dr. Oz went on to point out in this great magazine a little known side benefit to clean sinuses:

What a lot of people don't know is that the sinuses are linked closely to lung health. The sinuses are a major source of nitric oxide in the body. Nitric oxide opens things up: the blood vessels, the airways. When we intubate a patient through the nose, we always worry about how that will affect their breathing—because it can reduce the lungs' content of nitric oxide. So, it follows that keeping the sinuses healthy also keeps the lungs full of fresh clean air. We don't yet know whether nasal irrigation is as helpful for asthma as it is for sinus problems, but it certainly will do more good than harm for asthmatics.

It doesn't take a whole lot of nitric oxide to work either. When he says that it opens things up like the blood vessels and the airways he means that it lowers blood pressure because the arteries are more relaxed; it means the heart doesn't have to work as hard; and our own experience with the nasal spray eliminating asthma may be related to this relaxing effect. More specifically the reopening of the airway that we saw in our patient DC, who had the problem of airway remodeling that was thought to be permanent in chronic asthmatics, is just what we would expect if nitric oxide is put back in the mix.

When the world-renowned author and health lecturer Susan Smith Jones was almost 18, she learned about the healing power of neti—nasal cleansing—from her grandmother. At that time in her life, her diet was "deplorable" and she was rarely without allergies. She carried copious amounts of tissues with her everywhere to wipe her runny nose, deal with her sneezing and to take care of all the extra mucus that she was coughing up. "It was not a pretty picture and my physician apprised me that I would have to live with this condition the rest of my life," says the healthy living expert.

Then one day when she was visiting her grandmother, the older woman told her if she followed her healthful guidance and suggestions, she guaranteed that she not only would see her allergies and sinus problems clear up within 30 days but also her entire life would be improved. Along with a new diet of whole foods, deep breathing, visualization and meditation, her grandmother introduced her to neti.

Her grandma called it her "easy breathing" practice.

"She didn't have a neti pot; she used a small teapot with a spout. In less than four weeks of practicing nasal cleaning two times a day... I was free from excess mucus, allergies, sneezing, constant throat clearing, extra weight and a pessimistic attitude," recalls Susan. "And my grandmother went from being someone who was strange and weird to me with her 'health nut' approach to life, to my greatest mentor and the person who changed my life for the better."

Nasal irrigation with a neti was "effective" in reducing overall incidence of colds among practitioners, according to Dr. Richard Ravizza of Pennsylvania State University who presented the findings recently at the 50th Scientific Assembly of the American Academy of Family Physicians, held in San Francisco.

Ravizza and Dr. John Fornadley placed 294 college students into three groups. One performed nasal irrigation; another took placebo pills; the third was left untreated. The students kept a "cold symptoms diary."

The authors found that students who used the daily saline rinse experienced a significant reduction in the number of colds contracted compared with non-users. On average, those engaging in nasal irrigation had fewer colds over the study period, the authors say, compared with the placebo or untreated groups.

Most people mix their own saline solution and when done right there is no problem. But the tendency is "if a little works well, then more should work better." Jerry had sinus problems when she was a child, even having her sinuses operated on at age six. They didn't know about neti pots so she had to 'sniff' saline into her nose. Too much salt in this mixture and the cilia get paralyzed; and it damages other parts of the nose as well so she still can't smell unless the skunk is in the backyard.

There is another a caveat with neti pots. This has been looked at in a study that should calm my fears, but I still hesitate. Irrigation can be too vigorous and it washes out both good and bad bacteria. We no longer encourage women to douche because it washed out both good and bad bacteria; and opened them to more serious infections. I can't stop wondering if nasal irrigation does not do the same thing. The evidence and the experience seems to say no, and I am willing to watch and wait, but using our spray is a whole lot easier, and I think just as effective, if not more so; it just hasn't been around that long.

CHAPTER EIGHT

Dental Health

I can't resist turning to the topic of xylitol and dental health. I can promise you one more great benefit from using xylitol: far fewer cavities. Unlike so many of our medical drugs today, where almost all side effects are bad news, xylitol offers some terrific overall health benefits. This is really good news.

Beginning almost forty years ago in Finland, after people had been using it to replace sugar for some time, dental researchers there, knowing that sugar contributed to tooth decay, thought that xylitol might be a means of preventing that problem. The first study they did to check this out looked at the change in the amount of decay over a two-year test period in a number of people that was divided into three groups: one group used regular sugar to sweeten their diets, another used fructose, and a third used xylitol. The amount of tooth decay was measured before and after. Those that ate regular sugar had the most progress in decay, those that ate fructose had less, but those eating xylitol had none. This was the first of "Turku Sugar Studies."

In Finland, where the government provides health services, this was good news because prevention is almost always better and less expensive than treatment. But internationally approved drug laws still handicap the government from allowing the 'drug' claims that xylitol prevents tooth decay, so again relatively few people know. Fortunately the size of this first study was such that the people there were aware of it and they did something about it. When you go to a dentist in Finland you don't get a toothbrush, you get gum. The Finnish Health Ministry has had to be creative in letting their population know about the studies and supporting the schools in programs using xylitol.

After some further confirming studies the Finns started putting xylitol in chewing gum. Chewing gum is an excellent way to get xylitol to the teeth and an easy way to study dosing effects, and the overwhelming majority of the studies done since the 1970s have used gum. More than 30 years of such studies have shown that chewing two sticks of gum two or three times a day doesn't help much, but four times a day helps noticeably, and five times a day prevents about 80 percent of tooth decay.

There has also been enough time to do laboratory and clinical studies to find out how and why xylitol protects our teeth. These studies were also among the first to find out how tooth decay actually begins. First of all we have bacteria that live in our mouths and on our teeth. They make up the plaque on our teeth that the dental hygienist removes regularly when we have our teeth cleaned. This plaque is a biofilm, a home for these bacteria. Most of them are nice to us in that they don't infect us, but these researchers found that when many of the bacteria eat the sugars in our diets they make an acid that eats through the hard enamel surfaces of our teeth. This is how cavities begin. The particular bacteria that do the most damage are called *Streptococcus mutans* and studies on the preventive effects of xylitol have shown several significant effects of xylitol on this family of bacteria.

First of all they found that these bacteria eat xylitol thinking they can use it for food. But the bacteria lack the enzymes needed to digest five carbon sugars so they get indigestion; and not just simple indigestion because their structure is really distorted after they eat xylitol—it looks like they are literally writhing in agony. They also found that the bacteria did learn not to eat the xylitol; and, very nicely for us and our tooth decay, when they learned this they also learned not to make the acid any more. Remember the message of xylitol to the bacteria: to 'shape up or ship out.' This is an example of bacteria shaping up.

Other dental researchers have looked at what xylitol does to the biofilm on our teeth. Most recently studies done in France showed that xylitol impaired the ability of many cavity-causing bacteria to both make biofilm and the acid.

LONG-TERM PROTECTION

One of the more interesting of the dental studies looked at young children in Belize. This study was in two parts. The first part lasted two years and tested a variety of combinations of sugar alcohols in the gums. Sugar alcohols all work to replace the glucose or corn syrup in our diets and if that was the reason for the benefit they would all work equally well at reducing tooth decay. This and most of the other studies gave a significant edge to xylitol. There were no real surprises in the first part of this study with the xylitol only gum performing significantly better than the other options.

The second study was a follow-up, done five years later, with no exposure to xylitol in this interim, and there were surprises. Just as they did with all these studies, dentists look at the child's teeth and count the cavities before and after, comparing numbers in both cases. When they returned and counted cavities they found there was, as expected, more decay, but they also found that the permanent teeth, *which had erupted in the xylitol only group during the first two year long study, had 95 percent less decay than the other teeth.*

These children received a long-term benefit from chewing xylitol sweetened gum for two years. As we saw earlier long-term benefits are when a particular action leads to a benefit long after the action is finished. In a case involving a bacterial action such as tooth decay, long-term benefits mean that the bacteria have either gone away or changed to a different nature. The most reasonable guess for the particular benefit of the children in Belize is that the regular presence of xylitol while their permanent teeth were coming in led to a biofilm on those particular teeth that did not have any acid making bacteria. This is also the most likely reason for the benefits seen in the studies of children whose mothers chew this gum regularly that have been done by Eva Söderling and her group, also in Finland.

These children are never exposed to xylitol, but they have significantly fewer cavities at age five and counting than comparable children whose mothers do not chew xylitol gum. This benefit, like that of the children in Belize, likely comes from the fact that the biofilm on these teeth is established as they erupt and if cavity causing bacteria are not there at that time they can't get there later. In Belize they were prevented because the children were chewing xylitol gum; in Söderling's group they were prevented because the mothers' chewing of the gum spread helpful bacteria to their children.

NON-ACID ENVIRONMENT

This eruption time is critical for the proper development of tooth enamel. As new teeth emerge into the mouth, the enamel is somewhat soft and porous. A non-acidic environment with the proper minerals strengthens this new enamel. Conversely it can be easily damaged by an acid environment that eats through the soft enamel and keeps the needed minerals in solution; new teeth erupting into such an acidic environment are considered to be at higher risk for decay.

Xylitol can provide crucial benefits for newly erupting teeth. Proper xylitol use provides an ideal non-acidic environment, and xylitol acts as a carrier for calcium, which enhances the natural mineralization process. The combination of xylitol properties enables the new enamel to be optimally mineralized and provides long-term resistance to tooth decay.

TIMING IS IMPORTANT

There is a brief "window of opportunity" for a lasting protective effect when new teeth emerge through gum tissue. Ideally xylitol use should begin before the new tooth shows up, thereby setting ideal conditions to welcome in the new arrival.

Setting the Sage—Baby Teeth

The best way to prepare for a life of perfect teeth is to start at the beginning. Baby teeth ("primary teeth") are extremely important for the proper development and positioning of the permanent adult teeth. Decay can progress very rapidly through the thin enamel of the primary teeth. Tooth decay at a young age can lead to serious infections, as well as esthetic and orthodontic problems. Fortunately, early tooth decay is almost entirely preventable. Current recommendations include limiting the frequency of sugar consumption, especially between meals and before bedtime. But these are weak and poor considering what we know about how xylitol works.

Mothers should use xylitol to prevent transmission of acid making/decay causing bacteria to their infants; and they should start several months before the infant is born in order to shed the harmful bacteria prior to the time they expose their infants to these germs. Infants should use it to insure a proper environment. It's even available in a gel form that goes in a pacifier.

Ages 5 to 12

The transition period between baby teeth and permanent teeth is the "mixed dentition" time. For most children this occurs between the ages of 5 and 12. You may remember an advertising slogan referring to this time as "the cavity–prone years." This is when children start being able to satisfy their own sweet tooth and sugary products that do this are super abundant. Fortunately, because of the xylitol products we now have available, this "high-risk" period can now be regarded as "times of opportunity." There are lots of xylitol based candies, mints, and gums that will satisfy the child's desire for sugar as well as help their teeth develop; and there are lots of cookie recipes with xylitol. Xylitol at this time changes the eruption period to one of enhanced protection as demonstrated in the Belize study—95 percent less cavities in these erupted teeth.

GOAL

Our goal is to have healthy teeth with no decay and no fillings. We now have the added protection of xylitol as extra insurance at those times we need it most. With the help of xylitol, tooth eruption can now be regarded as a great opportunity to develop the best smile possible.

Here is the bottom line: Using xylitol in the form of mints, chewing gum and toothpaste can help:

- Reduce cavities by up to 80 percent
- Inhibit the ability of cavity-causing, plaque-forming bacteria to stick to teeth
- Reverse early cavity formation

PART OF AN OVERALL STRATEGY

The California Dental Association recommends patients consider xylitol "as part of an overall strategy for decay reduction" and adds that, "With xylitol use, the quality of the bacteria in the mouth changes and fewer and fewer decay-causing bacteria survive on tooth surfaces. Less plaque forms and the level of acids attacking the tooth surface is lowered."

Did you know your dental insurance plan may cover xylitol-based products? Oral xylitol is so effective some dental insurance plans provide members with discounts on products. See if such products are covered by your dental insurance plan, and if they aren't ask them why not. It is clear that using xylitol regularly is a very effective way of preventing tooth decay and that it works primarily because of an interaction with the bacteria that cause the decay. If you wish to prevent these problems in yourself and your children then use xylitol regularly. The U.S. military has recognized these benefits and now puts xylitol-sweetened gum in the packaged meals used by all of our military when they are deployed or in the field, but few of them are told what the gum is for. While there is a pamphlet available that explains the dental benefits of xylitol the only reason for including gum with their meals understood by the many service men and women we have asked is that it keeps them regular.

Catherine Hayes, of the Harvard Dental School wrote are review article on the beneficial effects of xylitol and other sugar alcohols in preventing tooth decay in which she said:

> Furthermore, since the evidence suggests a strong caries protective effect of xylitol it would be unethical to deprive subjects of its potential benefits. Given that several of the criteria for causality are met, it is concluded that xylitol can significantly decrease the incidence of dental caries. (emphasis added)

It is good that the U.S. military has the ethics to make xylitol available; it is lamentable that they don't talk more about it.

As with the spray, this is not a drug so drug regulations don't apply. This means that one can put very little xylitol in the gum yet still splash it all over the label. Again, check the ingredients list; if xylitol is not the first listed ingredient look for another product.

We've mentioned this earlier, but it needs to be remembered that xylitol is not absorbed as well as other sugars so more of it stays in the GI tract where it holds onto water. More water in the GI tract means looser stools. The soldiers we have talked with about the gum they are given know this, and many of them know it by experience. The gum tastes good, but too much gives you diarrhea. This is a very individual problem and your body does seem to learn. Most Finns do not report any problems with xylitol and those using it regularly do increase their tolerance. The up side of this is that putting a teaspoon or two in your coffee is a very good way to keep one regular—and it does.

HOW TO USE XYLITOL MOST EFFECTIVELY TO PREVENT TOOTH DECAY

- Look for xylitol-sweetened products that encourage chewing or sucking to keep the xylitol in contact with your teeth. Important: The best items use xylitol as the principal sweetener.
- Studies show that 4 to 12 grams of xylitol per day are very effective. So have a wide variety of xylitol products: chewing gum, mints, toothpaste, mouthwashes and rinses, sweeteners, and more.
- Remember, if used only occasionally or even as often as once a day, xylitol may NOT be effective, regardless of the amount. Use xylitol at least three, and preferably 5 times every day.
- It's easy to keep track of your xylitol intake. "All xylitol" mints and gums contain about one gram of xylitol in each piece. You could begin with as little as one piece four times a day for a total of four grams. It is not necessary to use more than 15 grams per day as higher intakes yield diminishing dental benefits.
- Brush with xylitol. Xylitol-based toothpastes should list xylitol as their first or second ingredient (after water). Some toothpaste brands provide both xylitol and fluoride. The two are complementary.

TIMING

- Use immediately after eating; and clear the mouth with water first. Between meals, replace ordinary chewing gum, breath mints, or breathe spray with comparable xylitol products.

ORTHODONTIC BENEFITS

Before leaving the subject of dental benefits we need to say a word about the likelihood of significant orthodontic benefits. I spoke at a conference on xylitol early in 2009 and when I finished an orthodontist present asked if my nasal use of xylitol would prevent one of the commonest and severest problems that he sees in his practice. He explained that infants and children who breathe through their mouths change the tension of the facial and jaw muscles so that the palate raises and the jaw narrows. I can attest to the frequency of this problem since both a grandson and Heather's father had this problem; and it requires long term head gear and braces to correct.

I hedged above when I said 'likelihood' because ear, nose and throat doctors think that this is not a developmental problem, but that the children are born that way. I tend to agree with the dentists on this because the individuals I know with the problem had serious nasal congestion when they were toddlers, and those children who have trouble nose breathing that I see in my practice are all able to breathe normally through the nose if it is kept clean.

While the argument has just begun on the causes of this problem it just adds to the reasons for keeping your nose clean. This is one that leads to major expenses with orthodontics, but it is not nearly as important as keeping the nose open to avail yourself of the defenses that are there. Mouth breathing bypasses nasal defenses as well as the conditioning effect of the nasal membranes in the air we breathe.

CHAPTER NINE

Health and Healing Protocols

One of the most interesting "side effects" of xylitol is that it offers so many "side benefits." I am going to give you my thoughts and quick prescriptions for xylitol and its intended uses, as well as some of these fabulous side benefits. Overall, your health will benefit when you put some xylitol into your diet.

I'll also tell you about additional nutritional strategies that might be helpful to support your health and healing progress. Please be sure to work with your own doctor as you incorporate these into your health program.

ACNE

Acne is a common problem in those years when hormones are blossoming. It comes from bacteria getting into the pores of the skin which are then blocked with the thick secretions these children have as their bodies learn how to exude smells that make them more appealing. I have seen significant success dealing with this problem when xylitol is used regularly in skin cleaning. Here as in elsewhere it seems to effect the bacteria that cause most problems.

Put a tablespoon in 4 ounces of a liquid soap solution and use regularly.

ALLERGIES

One more story. We have a friend whose life was controlled by her allergies. She lives in Abilene so we don't get to see her that often, but she called the other day and told how her life had changed; she hardly notices her problem anymore. She related that her physician husband had also recently begun to use the spray. She commented that he was a lot like Naaman, the Captain of the Syrian army who wouldn't go bathe seven times in the river Jordan, as Elisha recommended in order to cure his leprosy, because it was too simple. Simple it is—keep your nose clean.

ASTHMA

A few years ago our doorbell rang. It was our postal lady. She had been delivering our mail for some time and finally got up enough nerve to ask us if we were the people who had developed the nasal spray her husband had been using. We told her we were the guilty parties and she thanked us. Her husband had asthma and their lives for years had been controlled by his illness. Since he began using the spray we developed his asthma had disappeared and they can now travel and do what they want without having to consider the asthma. She said, "We got our lives back!" And so can anyone who is dealing with the problems we have been talking about. I only say this to reinforce my one big idea, one that works: *Again, the key is regular use of your nasal xylitol—four to five times daily—each time you wash your hands. It's that simple. Keep your nose clean.*

Of course, it is also vitally important that you or your child consume plenty of fresh fruits and vegetables, which are rich in antioxidants. Studies show clearly that incorporating these great foods into your diet can also be extremely helpful.

BRONCHITIS

Bronchitis is inflammation of the bronchi, the tubes that carry the air we breathe from the trachea into all of the different segments of the lungs. Almost always this is caused by bacteria or viruses that have first colonized the back of the nose and then gotten into the air that we breathe and into our respiratory passages because the mucus is dry enough that it doesn't hold them well enough to expel them. Mouth breathing also bypasses nasal defenses and increases the risk of bronchitis. Maintaining optimum nasal defenses with your xylitol—inhaled four to five times daily—is the best and easiest way to prevent bronchitis.

If you wish to supplement xylitol cleansing with herbs, certainly ivy leaf supplements are excellent for helping to relax the bronchial passages. They are used throughout Europe for this purpose and can be useful.

CANDIDA

Researchers report in an article, entitled "The influence of dietary carbohydrates on in vitro adherence of four Candida species to human buccal epithelial cells," published in 2005 in *Microbial Ecology in Health and Disease* (17;3:156-162) that consumption of xylitol may help control oral infections of Candida yeast by interfering with their colonization; in contrast, galactose, glucose, and sucrose may increase proliferation, according to the same article.

Mom and dad, try to nix the high-fructose juices too. Perhaps worst of all is a diet laced with high-fructose corn syrup as found in altogether too many kids' beverages and other types of junk food. For overall health, this is so important. Water, alkalized preferably, teas, and other non-sugar beverages are going to help improve your condition.

I recommend quality probiotic formulas. Probiotics are beneficial bacteria that help the body to maintain its defenses too, especially in the gut where three-quarters of your immune cells are manufactured.

CANCER PREVENTION

Here's an interesting one: instead of using aspartame or saccharin as a sweetener try a packet of xylitol. While saccharin and aspartame truly raise serious health issues, xylitol has only healthy "side benefits" as this chapter shows, and it would make a smart alternative to these other less healthy artificial sweeteners.

CAVITY PREVENTION

Preventing cavities is how xylitol began as a means of improving our health. Xylitol talks to our bacteria and tells them to shape up or ship out.

- Bacteria living on our teeth make acid from the sugars we eat and as that acid then eats into our teeth a cavity is born.

- Xylitol tells the bacteria to go away if they won't stop making the acid—and they do both in the end.

I strongly recommend that you brush with a xylitol-based toothpaste, chew xylitol gums, use xylitol breath mints, and use it in your cooking. The only thing it doesn't do is raise yeast. It might sound counter-intuitive because the mints themselves are delicious, but if you and your kids will eat these regularly, you will enjoy superb dental health.

Even try baking with xylitol. Plenty of informative cookbooks abound.

CONSTIPATION

People get concerned when their bowels don't work properly, and there are lots of options available to remedy this problem. But regular use of most of them introduces problems of their own. We should try to use the simplest and the safest when dealing with this problem. When my mother was put into hospice care they added daily doses of sorbitol to keep her bowels from stopping up. In hospice they rely on the safest and least expensive ways of maintaining bodily functions and making their patients comfortable, and this was just one example. Xylitol works in exactly the same way as sorbitol and costs less. The importance of adequate fluid intake is a critical part of all remedies for this problem. Try sweetening with a little xylitol.

CYSTIC FIBROSIS

Cystic fibrosis is a genetic condition that affects the defenses of the airway by hampering proper mucus. The mucus of children with cystic fibrosis is thick and not very moveable. Our spray helps this process and use of xylitol in an aerosol for administration in a nebulizer to the entire bronchial and pulmonary field in children with cystic fibrosis is the focus of the University of Iowa group as they pursue their patent on this use of xylitol.

Every child with this condition should use xylitol both nasally and by nebulizer several times a day.

But there is something else that helps as much or more according to an associate we have who has children of her own with this condition—and for anybody dealing with this condition, this is important. Political scientist and CF researcher Valerie M. Hudson tells the following story:

When our first child with cystic fibrosis (CF) was diagnosed in August 1997, I quickly dove into the medical literature despite the fact that my doctorate was in political science. I was determined to understand not only the disease itself, but also the then-current state of its treatment.

I was dismayed to discover that at that time, the emphasis was on reaction to decline, not prevention of decline. At this point, the CF research community was pursuing gene therapy as a complete cure. This is not true today in 2009, but the small molecule correctors and potentiators which are the new (and much more promising) research thrust are not due to be approved for clinical use for another five years or so.

So treatment consisted primarily of the mucolytic DNase plus albuterol to open airways for inhalation of DNase, plus all manner of IV, oral, and nebulized antibiotics and antifungals to deal with chronic respiratory infection. In addition, chest physical therapy (CPT) or other percussive therapy, was adjunct.

However, all of these treatments were double-edged swords for the patient. Classical CPT with postural drainage encouraged gastroesophageal reflux disease or GERD, which seeded respiratory infection. Physicians called into question the universal and daily use of albuterol even in infants. Some concerns were raised about DNase. The frequent use of antibiotics produced hyper-mutable drug-resistant strains of bacteria, while completely deranging gut flora.

Also of concern was the entire notion of a CF Clinic. In 1997, all CF patients would be asked to come into a hospital-based clinic, wait in the same waiting room, and use the same exam rooms with no serious disinfecting between patients. In other words, it was disastrous for the patients in terms of the spread of dangerous hyper-mutable strains of bacteria. Things have certainly improved since that time, with much stricter infection control and segregation of patients, but that CF 'clinics' still exist means we have a ways to go in terms of making CF care more rational.

So in 1997, our family was led to feel that there had to be a better way. This did not mean that we rejected all conventional CF treatment. Absolutely not. However, we felt strongly that there had to be harmless ways of strengthening the CF body to significantly reduce the velocity of decline.

In 1998, when new research appeared showing that reduced glutathione (GSH) was effluxed at the epithelial surface by the CFTR channel, we began to feel there might be a way to accomplish our objective. [The CFTR channel is the abbreviation for the cystic fibrosis transmembrane conductance regulator, which is associated with many cases of cystic fibrosis. The fact that this channel does not work properly in children with CF and that glutathione is what it releases when it is functioning properly is what Dr. Hudson honed in on. More information on it can be found at: http://student.biology.arizona.edu/honors97/group7/cftrpage.html (accessed 10/22/2009)]

The more we investigated the role of GSH, the more we were struck by the similarity between the effects of GSH deficiency in the extracellular milieu, on the one hand, and the symptomology of CF on the other. I wrote a peer-reviewed summary article on this comparison for Free Radical Biology and Medicine in 2001.

Knowing that GSH was readily available as a nutritional supplement, we determined to get GSH into our son and see if it made a difference. We used both oral GSH (with and without co-factors), and buffered nebulized GSH. We began this regimen in the autumn of 1998.

We saw outstanding results. Weight gain, always difficult for those with CF, no longer was an issue. Our son, the 5th percentile for weight at the time of his diagnosis, soon reached the 95th percentile for weight. He developed a ravenous appetite. He kicked his staph infection. He began to drool for the first time. His snot was no longer of Super Glue consistency. Those who have children with CF will recognize how significant these changes are. And the changes continued: for example, when our family gets sick, it is our CF children who recover the quickest.

We now have three children with CF who culture nothing, are all above the 50th percentile for weight, have normal liver enzymes, and have normal blood sugar.

We use much more than GSH with our children. However, we consider GSH to be the main pillar of our approach, which we will continue to use until these small molecule correctors and potentiators come on line. GSH has toned down the inflammation of their gut and lungs. It has served as a potent mucolytic. It has strengthened their immune system and made it more effective. We believe that the rate of decline of our CF children has been significantly diminished.

Our insurance company should also be very pleased. Cost of care for CF patients is normally extraordinarily high. But our children—aside from our first child's hospitalization on the eve of diagnosis with Pseudo-Bartter's Syndrome—have not had to be hospitalized, have not had to use expensive antibiotics or expensive mucolytics.

Finally, GSH is not only completely non-toxic, but is commonly used as an anti-toxin in medical practice. There is no overdose level for GSH; it is that harmless. GSH has therefore not been a double-edged sword for our children— it has but a single edge, fighting the deterioration that CF creates. Fortunately, the CF research community is slowly but surely beginning to look more closely at GSH: there have been two clinical trials of GSH use in CF, and there are two more underway. Hopefully the benefits of GSH therapy will one day be more broadly recognized.

CHEILITIS (ANGULAR CHEILITIS)

Angular cheilitis is a condition caused by a fungal infection in the corners of the lips that causes them to crack and bleed. It is more common in older people, especially those with dentures.

Chewing xylitol sweetened gum has been shown to help this process.

DIABETES

Diabetes rates are skyrocketing. I see many more pre-diabetics with a constellation of symptoms doctors call Syndrome X that consist of obesity, hypertension, high cholesterol and triglycerides, and other symptoms of heart disease.

Diabetes is the inability to deal adequately with glucose, the primary source of energy for most animals. The problem is either the inability to produce insulin (type 1 diabetes) or for insulin to be effective (type 2 diabetes).

In both cases dietary xylitol may help. In fact, xylitol was originally used as a safe all-natural alternative to sugar among diabetics.

Possessing approximately 40 percent less food energy, xylitol is absorbed more slowly than sugar and doesn't contribute to high blood sugar levels or the resulting hyperglycemia caused by insufficient insulin response. In this way, cooking and sweetening with xylitol makes sense.

Introducing xylitol should be done slowly so that the body can increase those enzyme systems and pathways that metabolize it rather than leaving it in the gut where it increases diarrhea.

The body metabolizes xylitol and other five carbon sugars in what is called the pentose monophosphate shunt where the end product is glucagon, which is easily turned into glucose in the cells. Glucagon is often used in diabetics who are hypoglycemic (low in their blood glucose levels) because it provides ready access to glucose, when it is needed, without raising the glucose levels. For brittle diabetics who have problems with frequent low blood sugar, having adequate glucagon stores is an obvious benefit.

Add to this the fact that xylitol has the same sweetness as sugar yet has a third fewer calories and its benefits are even more clear. Yet that is not all. Many people with type 2 diabetes have found that a low glycemic diet helps them better deal with their condition. They rely on what has come to be known as the glycemic index, which measures how much a specific amount (usually 100 grams) of a specific food raises glucose levels. The purpose of this is to decrease the glucose load with which these people must deal. Critics point out that people don't eat single foods and that the index doesn't deal with combinations of foods as they are more often served, but any effort to decrease the challenge of glucose to these people is a benefit. And the glycemic index of xylitol is a paltry 7, meaning it hardly has any effect on blood glucose.

Again with juvenile type 1 diabetes, xylitol is a wonderful addition to the diet, for use as a sweetener. It can only be of benefit to any child coping with juvenile onset of diabetes.

EAR INFECTIONS (OTITIS MEDIA)

For ear infections, of course, you will want to give your child xylitol nasally five times a day, as a preventive, and during any prescribed treatment courses. Pediatricians have been warned repeatedly to cut down on antibiotic use but more and more recommend xylitol too as a means of taking a proactive approach. I hope that with publication of this book many more pediatricians will get their earache patients using xylitol. It would be so good for reducing our number of special education students and help us to avoid overuse of antibiotics and ventilation tubes. Remember, if your child goes to day care or school you will need the help of their day care workers and teachers most likely if they are not able to wash their noses with xylitol spray.

FLU

Influenza or flu is best prevented with the regular use of Xylitol. Both use of intranasal xylitol and xylitol with the neti pot would be excellent preventive measures. Whenever you travel during cold and flu season be sure to wash your nose with xylitol. Do it every time you wash your hands. Keeping your nose flushed with xylitol and moisture will help to eliminate the threat at the source. Also do the same daily for work situations.

Xylitol should also be used if you contract the flu—try to avoid, unless critical, the use of antihistamines and decongestants, as in the long run, these will compromise your immune defenses, especially the nasal defenses. On the other hand, the use of nasal xylitol will help to improve the defenses and aid in recovery time.

GAS

Intestinal gas comes from the bacterial breakdown of what we eat. Eating xylitol decreases the material the bacteria eat and reduces gas. Gums, mints, and baking with xylitol will all help with this problem. I recommend taking a probiotic regularly to help too.

HEART DISEASE

I was working in an ER some time ago when one of our nurses was brought in by ambulance in the middle of a heart attack. He had not worked in the ER for the past few days because he was home with a respiratory illness. We took prompt care of his heart and he survived, but this experience joggled other memories of an association between cardiac events and upper respiratory conditions. We touched on this when we commented on Dr. Oz's discussion of the importance of nitric oxide and how it relaxes things, including the blood vessels and the lungs. Relaxing these things in particular reduces the burden on the heart and if opening your sinuses where nitric oxide is made and released can help then we should. But there is another way that xylitol can be useful. Definitely linked to heart disease are high rates of infectious organisms in your pipes, the arteries and vessels that carry your blood, and also in your mouth. In other words, poor oral health usually is associated with poor heart and circulatory health. Take care of your nasal defenses and dental health to help maintain heart and circulatory health. Again, when we think of our defenses against these organisms, the upper respiratory passages come to mind. By reducing the bacterial build-up in two of the key entry points, our nasal passages and our mouths, we are definitely improving our health. So all things xylitol are good for your heart: chew xylitol gum, enjoy the breath mints, and even considering sweetening and baking with it.

HYPOGLYCEMIA

Low blood sugar is a problem for many diabetics and even some normal people. It is caused by increases in insulin secretion that drop the glucose levels by enough that symptoms are produced. The reason that xylitol helps this condition are discussed above under diabetes.

IMMUNE HEALTH

Xylitol positively impacts the immune system and seems to awaken the body's white blood cells much like other positively acting long and short chain sugars (polysaccharides). In rats, xylitol has been found to increase the activity of the white blood cells called neutrophils that are involved in fighting off bacteria; a benefit has even been seen during sepsis or blood infection, according to a May 11, 2008 report from Marjo Renko and co-investigators in *BMC Microbiology* (8:45).

MASTOIDITIS AND MENINGITIS

Mastoiditis is an infection in the mastoid bones that are next to the middle ear and they generally begin by extension from the middle ear. If this infection is not recognized promptly and surgically drained it commonly opens and drains into the brain causing meningitis or infection in the brain and you don't want this. Again these bacteria most commonly begin in the back of the nose. Even epidemic meningitis, caused by the bacteria

Neisseria meningitidis, begins in the nose. Dealing with this specific problem is only on my wish list, because the idea of washing these bacteria from the nose is too new to have any research looking at this benefit. So again washing your nose with xylitol would be really smart if meningitis infections occur in your areas. Occasionally, we see clusters at universities and in communities.

OSTEOPOROSIS
Xylitol also appears to have potential for help with osteoporosis. Dietary xylitol prevents weakening of bones in biological models and improves bone density. Again, cooking with xylitol and using it as a sweetener just makes a lot of sense.

PREGNANT OR NURSING WOMEN
Xylitol studies show that regular use significantly reduces the probability of transmitting the Streptococcus mutans bacteria, which is responsible for tooth decay, from mother to child during the first two years of life and that such kids have far fewer dental caries. Xylitol mints and chewing gum and even sweetening with xylitol are all on the world's safe and recommended lists.

Xylitol has no known toxicity in humans, and people have consumed as much as 400 grams daily for long periods with no apparent ill effects. Women may safely use xylitol during pregnancy (inform your doctor).

When obstructive sleep apnea occurs because of nasal obstruction then by all means keep the nose clean. For dealing with complete obstruction see the section on using neti pots at the end of chapter 8.

OBESITY
Calories play a part in most weight loss programs and if you have sweet tooth xylitol has the same sweetness but a third fewer calories than sugar.

NASAL POLYPS
Nasal polyps are almost always a response to local irritants and removing those irritants should prevent them. They are currently treated with nasal

steroids, which turn off the immune system so it doesn't recognize the irritants, or with surgery. We feel it better to prevent them in the first place, but even when they are there the concentration of xylitol in the spray we use is greater than that of the fluid in the polyp and regular and frequent use should shrink them; and removing the irritants by the regular cleaning removes the stimulus for their development in the first place. KEEP YOUR NOSE CLEAN!

PEDIATRIC FEBRILE SEIZURES

Febrile seizures are a major concern of parents, but are not a medical problem. If one is certain that the seizure is only due to fever the advice of my pediatrics professor is appropriate: "for heavens sake, don't just do something, stand there."

The problem is that there are many other causes of seizures and while they all look the same many of them need further workup. Febrile children less than 6 months of age do not have an adequately developed immune system and always should be taken to the doctor. Febrile children over six months should be supported and made comfortable. Remember that a fever is part of your inflammatory response and is there because it provides a survival benefit. Don't rush to treat it. (But do seek appropriate medical attention.)

The association of aspirin treated fevers due to viral infections and the subsequent development of Reyes Syndrome has switched the emphasis to using acetaminophen, but in the animal studies any lowering of fever with drugs in these artificially infected animals meant that more of them died. Maintaining adequate fluid intake is the most critical part of treating a fever so oral rehydration is important to remember, but anything the child will drink should be used.

Whether or not a person becomes sick with an infection depends on the virulence and amount of the infecting agent(s), and the defenses of the host. Using the concepts presented here we should be able to augment those defenses and reduce, if not eliminate, much of this problem.

PNEUMONIA

The respiratory syncytial virus picks especially on small children and it can lead to pneumonia. A common problem following these infections is the development of asthma. Our grandchildren have regularly attended day care for the past twelve years and have escaped numerous epidemics where many of the children have been infected with this virus and the only difference has been the regular use of the nasal spray. So for all kids, this is very smart preventive medicine. You just really do cut down on a lot of potential problems you see other kids having. You wish you could help them too. But you can by setting the example at your day care center.

SINUS PROBLEMS

Sinus infections are the adult counterpart to childhood ear infections. Back in the days before I went to medical school there were books published on coping with bleeding and blood clotting disorders of the newborn. Then someone discovered that giving the newborn a shot of vitamin K eliminated them. Now the books just gather dust. Sinus problems will have a similar fate if we will just keep our noses clean. Wash your nose four to five times daily for best results.

TINNITUS

Tinnitus is a constant ringing in the ears. It can be a side effect of taking some drugs, but more commonly results from recurrent ear infections that affect the middle ear. Again, keeping your nose clean reduces these infections and should reduce the tinnitus.

URINARY TRACT INFECTIONS

We discussed UTIs in the chapter on warfare with bacteria. Chronic UTIs should be treated with mannose or cranberry juice extracts for long enough to trade out the GI bacteria that cause this problem. By all means if you can identify a practice, such as bathing, that may contribute to their recurrence try to adapt in a way that helps prevent the self infection (a notable cause). Use of xylitol as a sweetener and in baking should also help, as will brushing with it, and using chewing gum.

VIRUSES

While the use of xylitol or other sugars is not associated with reducing viral adherence the washing is beneficial at reducing the viral load and this helps the immune system deal with it more effectively.

WOUNDS

Wounds usually heal without problems in a healthy population, but when a person has diabetes, or circulatory problems they become major problems. Wounds in diabetics feet generally led to amputation a few years ago. Hyperbaric oxygen helped preserve many, feet and legs from being amputated; and since many died within a few years of being amputated, it has helped many.

Randy Wolcott, a wound care physician in Lubbock, Texas, began experimenting with xylitol after we discussed its possible role in reducing biofilm adherence. Combining xylitol with lactoferrin he was able to increase the healing rate of ischemic wounds, like those of diabetics or people with poor circulation, from 65 percent to 77 percent. If you know someone with this problem you can find out more about Dr. Wolcott's methods at the Southwest Regional Wound Care Center in Lubbock, Texas or at their web site http://woundcarecenter.net/.

YEAST INFECTIONS

When I first learned about xylitol and went searching for it I found it at my local health food store where it had been recommended for ages as a treatment and preventive for yeast infections. These infections are common in people with too much glucose and using xylitol helped them to reduce that load while still savoring the sweet taste. (See also Candida.)

CHAPTER TEN

Putting it All Together

While upper airway problems are the most common reason for going to the doctor they are certainly not the only problems we have. Nor are our airway defenses the only ones we should be honoring and supporting.

Our bodies are living systems that adapt to the environments in which we live. Sometimes we change the environment to make us more comfortable and compromise the adaptations we have made in the past, like we do with our central heating and air conditioning and our nose's defenses.

Sociologists have looked at groups of healthy people and found that they share what Aaron Antonovsky, one of their leaders, calls a sense of coherence with their environment and their condition. Their environment is meaning- ful to them, it is not hostile; they have a greater sense of understanding their environment, and they feel that it is manageable. In other words, as we put it, it's something they are comfortable playing with.

We can learn a lot here from the bacteria. When they are threatened they adapt by developing resistance in order to survive. When they are not threat- ened they adapt toward living with the current environment; survival is not an issue so they adapt toward diversity and cooperation. This is the kind of adaptation we want to promote and we can do that by making the adapting agent more comfortable as they play with the elements in their environments.

This work, and this book, is the result of chronic ear infections, but peo- ple can and do adapt to these problems. Jerry was discussing the problems of chronic ear infections with a very successful and intelligent woman recently. When Jerry explained to her that one of the long-term problems of chronic ear infections was frequent mispronunciation, tears welled in the lady's eyes. She whispered that she herself had that problem, and that even though she was successful and respected in her profession, it had handicapped her whole life because she didn't take advantage of the many opportunities she had to talk because of her own embarrassment.

The educational facilities to deal with these problems are now available in our special education programs: speech therapy and classroom and teacher modifications. The problem is that children who require these services are often labeled slow learners and that label is seen as a threat to many children and their caring parents. It often prompts a defensive response that leads to each side digging in their heels as they argue over how to treat the child. More often these are handicapped children that can be rehabilitated; they are not slow and labeling them so does no good at all. Of course, the best way to deal with these problems now is to prevent them.

Jerry too, when she recently read about many of the residual problems of early ear infections, like the preference for silence, tone deafness, problems with syllables, and the same problem with pronunciation that plagued the life of the lady mentioned above, realized that her childhood ear infections had also left their mark. Penicillin was not readily available in the war years when Jerry experienced her problems, so her father comforted her by blowing smoke in her ears, without realizing, of course, that the secondhand smoke he was blowing in her face was a likely cause of her problem. But we do adapt, and when the environment is a loving one, with caring others blowing smoke in your ears to comfort you, those adaptations are more likely to be creative and toward wholeness because we are more comfortable playing with the elements in our environment when they are not threatening us.

Such play is more productive when it is informed and it would be best if you could find a physician willing to work with you, but there is enough information out there that you can usually educate yourself as well as relying on your physician; and as stated earlier you might have better luck with your local biologist. Dental hygienists, the people in your dentist's office that clean your teeth, are increasingly filling this role when it comes to keeping your teeth healthy, but there are few counterparts in the medical area.

Naturopathic physicians do this and recent additions to chiropractic education enable it as well. If you can find someone in your community with this kind of education build a relationship with them.

Ask them if thy have read this book and what they think of it.

The play needs to be informed; it should not be a response to pain or other perceived threats, which could lead to the use of drugs and/ or alcohol. Play that is a response to a threat or fear leads to resistance, which is not what you want since it is not creative. Creative play comes, again, with a sense of coherence—the condition is meaningful, manageable, and understandable. The tools for this creative play come from food and other materials—herbs, supplements, homeopathics, mind-body work, and others— usually covered under the category of alternative medicine.

By far the best advice I have ever seen dealing with the food we eat is from T. Colin Campbell's *The China Study*. In his book he reports the results of the largest study relating food and health that has ever been done, and he comes down hard with the conclusion that our diets are far better if they are based on plant foods that are minimally processed. I would also add to his information, though I do it more in principle than with any evidence, that the more variety and diversity one can get in their food the more likely they are to get the nutrients they need to be healthy. That is advice as well for the farmers that grow our food; monoculture is risky since it makes it so much easier for pests to eliminate the entire crop. Almost as revealing as Dr. Campbell's dietary recommendations is his recounting of the hassles he has had to go through with the American food industry in his talking about what he has determined to be a healthier way of eating in his broad and in depth study.

Read *The China Study* and play with your diet. Those dealing with food allergies point out that one needs to follow a diet for at least a week before one sees an effect. Sometimes it's faster. Jerry had juvenile rheumatoid arthritis when she was younger. She got markedly better when she went on a prolonged fast; she played with her diet. And she is not alone; other people with arthritis have seen similar benefits. She also found that avoiding red meat helps with her persistent whole body aches; and found this out after only two or three days on a cleansing diet.

And critically important in our play with food is including a wide variety of fruits and vegetables, preferably organic.

The sense of coherence that Antonovsky sees as critical in moving toward increased health, and the ability to play creatively with the elements in our environments, means that with creative play even how things fit together is open to adaptation; the goal is living in harmony with nature more than we have done.

I hope in this book that tens of thousands more children and adults alike will find that they can breathe easy and live lives free of allergies, asthma, sinus problems, middle ear infections, and so many other URIs that plague us, not by taking a heavy handed approach with our biggest guns and artillery (drugs and surgery) but by taming our enemy, keeping them subdued, outsmarting them in the end with superior ideas and methods. I try to make things simple for my patients and for all of you who have come to this book out of frustration and even desperation for help. It really is simple. I just go back to those caring words from my mom so long ago: "Keep your nose clean."

Resources

Quality xylitol formulas are available at health food stores, natural pharmacies, dental offices, retailers and from other health professionals under brand names such as Xlear and Spry. Visit www.xlear.com for more information.

Also visit www.xylitol.org and www.nasal-xylitol.com.

twitter For social media visit www.twitter.com/xylitolcure and www.twitter.com/xylitolinfo.

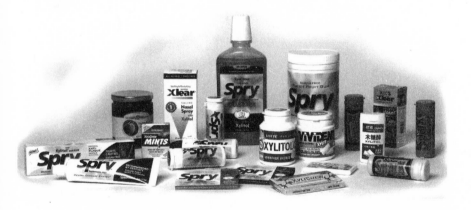

Oral Rehydration

Who should use it?

Anyone who needs to replace fluids or who needs a little extra fluid because of illness, such as the fever discussed above. Definitely people with gastrointestinal losses should use this; that is what it is designed for. Whenever someone is ill an IV will usually make them feel better. This is an IV you can drink. Pregnant women with nausea and vomiting can usually tolerate this and it prevents the dehydration that is usually treated with an IV. Extra fluid is always helpful when one is dealing with infection—it helps the washing. I have even used this successfully with diabetics who are vomiting, but vomiting diabetics can have serious problems and should be in a hospital.

Should anyone not use it?

People with heart disease can get too much fluid and develop what is called congestive heart failure. Oral rehydration is not a good idea for them. If a person has an ulcer that is perforating the wall of their stomach they will have a whole lot of pain and their stomach will be rigid. Putting anything in a stomach with holes is not wise.

How is it made?

Combine:

- 1 quart water,
- 3/4 teaspoon salt substitute (read the little print on the package, this should be mostly potassium chloride),
- 1/2 teaspoon baking soda, and
- 3 tablespoons white corn syrup (eg. Karo).

For other than babies this may be flavored with juice concentrate or unsweetened powdered drink mix such as Kool-Aid.

Important warning: measure the baking soda and salt substitute carefully to prevent imbalance problems.

How should it be used?

Some people chug-a-lug it, but this is not recommended. Best is to think of it as an IV and drink small amounts regularly. The journal *Pediatrics* (1984 Nov;74(5 Pt 2):950-4.) in an article by LS Book entitled "Vomiting and Diarrhea" recommends the following steps for infants that can easily be adapted upward for older people:

- *Step 1.* Wait one hour after the last episode of vomiting.
- *Step 2.* Give 1/2 oz. (15cc) to an infant or 1 oz. (30cc) to a child over one year old every 20 minutes for one to two hours. If an infant is being breast fed only two feedings of oral rehydration are all that is usually necessary.
- *Step 3.* If vomiting does not recur, increase the amount gradually. The goal is to replace the fluids lost within six hours. If vomiting does return go back to step 1.

  If you have gone through this cycle three times go to the doctor.
- *Step 4.* Advance the diet and resume normal diet in 12 to 24 hours.

Pay attention to your body; don't force anything on it that doesn'9t feel right. When you are adequately hydrated your body will know.

Why use this?

In this day when we can stop diarrhea with a pill and calm an upset stomach with a shot why should one go through the turmoil? The best answer is to trust your immune system and try to support it in what it feels is best for your body. Some people whose diarrhea is caused by bacteria become carriers of those harmful bacteria when their diarrhea is stopped with medication. Some children have died of infection when they were given medicine that stopped their diarrhea. Trust your body.

Endnotes

INTRODUCTION

Harold Magoun Jr, DO, FAAO, FCA, DO, ED (Hon). "More About the Use of OMT During Influenza Epidemics," published in *The Journal of the American Osteopathic Association*, October 2004, 104;10:406-407.

CHAPTER 2

The initial study on oral rehydration is: Sack RB, Cassells J, Mitra R, et al. The use of oral replacement solutions in the treatment of cholera and other severe diarrhoeal disorders. *Bull World Health Organ.* 1970; 43(3): 351-60.

The Lancet editors speak of oral rehydration as one of the most significant medical advances of the 20th Century in: Water with sugar and salt. *Lancet.* 1978 Aug 5; 2(8083): 264.

Anna Meinild and her colleagues explained how oral rehydration works in: Meinild A, Klaerke DA, Loo DD, Wright EM, Zeuthen T. The human Na+-glucose cotransporter is a molecular water pump. *J Physiol.* 1998 Apr 1; 508(Pt 1): 15-21.

Its lamentable use in the United States is reported in: Reis EC, Goepp JG, Katz S, Santosham M. Barriers to the use of oral rehydration therapy. *Pediatrics.* 1994 May; 93(5): 708-11.

Luotonen M, Uhari M, Aitola L, Lukkaroinen AM, Luotonen J, Uhari M, Korkeamaki RL. Recurrent otitis media during infancy and linguistic skills at the age of nine years. *Pediatr Infect Dis J.* 1996 Oct;15(10): 854-8.

Bennett KE, Haggard MP, Silva PA, Stewart IA. Behaviour and developmental effects of otitis media with effusion into the teens. *Arch Dis Child* 2001 Aug;85(2): 91-5.

The study showing that tubes do not help reverse hearing problems is: Lous J, Burton MJ, Felding JU, et al. Grommets (ventilation tubes) for hearing loss associated with otitis media with effusion in children. *Cochrane Database Syst Rev.* 2005 Jan 25; (1): CD001801.

The study showing the benefits of chewing gum for ear infections was: Uhari M. et al. Xylitol chewing gum in prevention of otitis media. *British Medical Journal.* 1996 Nov 9; 313(7066): 1180-84.

The safety of xylitol when it is put into the airway was studied by the group at the University of Iowa: Durairaj L, Launspach J, Watt JL, et al. Safety assessment of inhaled xylitol in mice and healthy volunteers. *Respir Res.* 2004 Sep 16;5:13.

The metaphor of dendritic connections as pathways that become roads and highways as they are used more and myelinated comes from personal conversations (pillow talk) with Jerry Bozeman, an expert in this area of childhood development.

The two articles in *Medical Hypotheses* are: Why the Increases in Upper Respiratory Infections? (2001 Sep;57(3):378-81.) and; The next step in infectious disease: taming bacteria. (2003 Feb;60(2):171-4).

CHAPTER 3

Christine Rogers study on environmental reasons for increased allergy was done with Gilmour MI, Jaakkola MS, London SJ, and Nel AE. How exposure to environmental tobacco smoke, outdoor air pollutants, and increased pollen burdens influences the incidence of asthma. *Environ Health Perspect.* 2006 Apr;114(4):627-33.

The study done in the Netherlands looking at the effect of allergies and the medicine used to treat them on learning was done by Vuurman EF, van Veggel LM, Uiterwijk MM, Leutner D, and O'Hanlon JF. Seasonal allergic rhinitis and antihistamine effects on children's learning. *The Annals of Allergy,* (1993 Aug;71(2):121-6).

Resa Aslan's book, *How to Win A Cosmic War*, (Random House. 2009) applies to our war on terrorism, but it is just as applicable to our war with bacteria. Bacteria and nation-states are at the extremes of living systems that are better seen and dealt with as complex adaptive systems, what we call CASYs in our book *The Boids and the Bees*, where this issue is better explained.

Starfield B. Is US health really the best in the world? *JAMA.* 2000 Jul 26;284(4): 483-5.

Schappert SM. Office visits for otitis media: United States, 1975-90. *Adv Data.* 1992 Sep 8; (214):1-19.

One article showing the differences in asthma between the developed world and Eastern European countries is: Priftanji A, Strachan D, Burr M, Sinamati J, Shkurti A, Grabocka E, Kaur B, Fitzpatrick S. Asthma and allergy in Albania and the UK. *Lancet,* 2001 Oct 27;358(9291):1426-7.

The CDC study of asthma prevalence is: Mannino DM, Homa DM, Pertowski CA, Ashizawa A, Nixon LL, Johnson CA, Ball LB, Jack E, Kang DS. Surveillance for asthma—United States, 1960-1995. *MMWR CDC Surveill Summ.* 1998 Apr 24; 47(1): 1-27. Data for our graph is taken from their Table 1.

Crater DD, Heise S, Perzanowski M, Herbert R, Morse CG, Hulsey TC, Platts-Mills T. Asthma hospitalization trends in Charleston, South Carolina, 1956 to 1997: twenty-fold increase among black children during a 30-year period. *Pediatrics 2001* Dec; 108(6): E97

Copeland AR. An assessment of lung weights in drowning cases. The Metro Dade County experience from 1978 to 1982. *Am J Forensic Med Pathol.* 1985 Dec;6(4):301-4.

The data on the agricultural use of antibiotics is taken from a monograph done by The Union of Concerned Scientists. *Hogging It: Estimates of Antimicrobial Abuse in Livestock*, by Margaret Mellon, Charles Benbrook, and Karen Lutz Benbrook, Union of Concerned Scientists, January 2001 (report available at http://www.ucsusa.org/).

The study from Turku, Finland showing participation and likely cooperation between both bacteria and viruses is: Ruohola A, Meurman O, Nikkari S, Skottman T, Salmi A,Waris M, Osterback R, Eerola E, Allander T, Niesters H, Heikkinen T, Ruuskanen O. Microbiology of acute otitis media in children with tympanostomy tubes: prevalences of bacteria and viruses. *Clin Infect Dis.* 2006 Dec 1;43(11):1417-22. Epub 2006 Oct 31.

Chris Post leads the Pittsburg researchers in looking at the role of biofilm in otitis. Post JC. Direct evidence of bacterial biofilms in otitis media. *Laryngoscope.* 2001 Dec;111[12]:2083-94.

Luanne Hall-Stoodley, PhD, Fen Ze Hu, PhD, Armin Gieseke, PhD, Laura Nistico, PhD, Duc Nguyen, PhD, Jay Hayes, BS, Michael Forbes, MD, David P. Greenberg, MD, Bethany Dice, BS, Amy Burrows, BS, P. Ashley Wackym, MD, Paul Stoodley, PhD, J. Christopher Post, MD, PhD, Garth D. Ehrlich, PhD, and Joseph E. Kerschner, MD. Direct Detection of Bacterial Biofilms on the Middle-Ear Mucosa of Children With Chronic Otitis Media." *JAMA.* 2006 July 12; 296(2): 202–211. Their results are worth repeating:

> Of the 26 children undergoing tympanostomy tube placement, 13 (50%) had OME [otitis media with effusion], 20 (77%) had recurrent OM [otitis media], and 7 (27%) had both diagnoses; 27 of 52 (52%) of the ears had effusions, 24 of 24 effusions were PCR-positive for at least 1 OM pathogen, and 6 (22%) of 27 effusions were culture-positive for any pathogen. Mucosal biofilms were visualized by CLSM [confocal laser scanning microscopy] on 46 (92%) of 50 MEM [middle ear mucosa] specimens from children with OME and recurrent OM using generic and pathogen-specific probes. Biofilms were not observed on 8 control MEM specimens obtained from the patients undergoing cochlear implantation.

Rayner MG, Zhang Y, Gorry MC, Chen Y, Post JC, Ehrlich GD. Evidence of bacterial metabolic activity in culture-negative otitis media with effusion. *JAMA.* 1998 Jan 28;279(4):296-9.

Ammons MC, Ward LS, Fisher ST, Wolcott RD, James GA. In vitro susceptibility of established biofilms composed of a clinical wound isolate of Pseudomonas aeruginosa treated with lactoferrin and xylitol. *Int J Antimicrob Agents.* 2009 Mar;33(3):230-6. Epub 2008 Nov 1.

CHAPTER 4

Profet M. The function of allergy: immunological defense against toxins. *Q Rev Biol.* 1991 Mar;66(1):23-62.

The asthma conference was the Keystone Symposium, which was held in Santa Fe, NM, February 2002.

Elliott MA, Sisson JH, Wyatt TA. Effects of cigarette smoke and alcohol on ciliated tracheal epithelium and Inflammatory Cell Recruitment. *Am J Respir Cell Mol Bio.* 2007 Apr; 36(4):452-9.

Rogers DF. Airway goblet cells: responsive and adaptable front-line defenders. *Europ Respiratory J,* 1994, Sep; 7(9):1690-706.

Svensson C, Andersson M, Grieff L, Persson CG. Nasal mucosal endorgan hyperresponsiveness. *American Journal of Rhinology,* 1998, Jan-Feb; 12(1):37-43.

CHAPTER 5

Arundel AV, Sterling EM, Biggin JH, Sterling TD. Indirect health effects of relative humidity in indoor environments. *Environ Health Perspect.* 1986 Mar;65:351-61.

Edwards DA, Man JC, Brand P, Katstra JP, et al. Inhaling to mitigate bioaerosols. *PNAS* Dec. 14, 2004, 101(50):17383-388.

Silber G, Proud D, Warner J, et al. In vivo release of inflammatory mediators by hyperosmolar solutions. *Am Rev Respir Dis.* 1988 Mar;137(3):606-12.

Kontiokari T, Uhari M, Koskela M. Antiadhesive effects of xylitol on otopathogenic bacteria, *J Antimicrob Chemother.* 1998 May;41(5):563-5.

Nathan Sharon and Halina Lis, Carbohydrates in Cell Recognition, *Scientific American,* January, 1993.

Ofek I, Goldhar J, Zafriri D, et al. Anti-Escherichia coli adhesion activity of cranberry and blueberry juices, *NEJM.* 1991 May 30;324(22):1599.

Zafriri D, Ofek I, Adar R, Pocino M, Sharon N, Inhibitory activity of cranberry juice on adherence of type 1 and type P fimbriated Escherichia coli to eucaryotic cells, *Antimicrob Agents Chemother* 1989 Jan;33(1):92-8.

Kontiokari T, Sundqvist K, Nuutinen M, Pokka T, Koskela M, Uhari M, Randomised trial of cranberry-lingonberry juice and Lactobacillus GG drink for the prevention of urinary tract infections in women, *BMJ* 2001 Jun 30;322(7302):1571-76.

Naaber P, Lehto E, Salminen S, Mikelsaar M. Inhibition of adhesion of Clostridium difficile to Caco-2 cells. *FEMS Immunol Med Microbiol.* 1996 Jul;14(4):205-9.

Akiyama H, Oono T, Huh WK, Yamasaki O, Ogawa S, Katsuyama M, Ichikawa H, Iwatsuki K. Actions of farnesol and xylitol against *Staphylococcus aureus. Chemotherapy.* 2002 Jul;48(3):122-8.

Durairaj L, Neelakantan S, Launspach J,Watt JL, Allaman MM, Kearney WR, Veng-Pedersen P, Zabner J. Bronchoscopic assessment of airway retention time of aerosolized xylitol. *Respir Res.* 2006 Feb 16;7:27

Zabner J, Seler MP, Launspach JL et al. The osmolyte xylitol reduces the salt concentration of airway surface fluid and may enhance bacterial killing. *Proceedings of the National Academy of Sciences USA.* 2000 Oct 10;97(21):11614-9.

CHAPTER 6

David Satcher, M.D., Ph.D. Emerging Infections: Getting Ahead of the Curve. *Emerging Infectious Disease,* Jan-Mar 1995; 1(1):1-6.

The dominance of bacteria in the scale of living organisms is from: Stephen J. Gould ed. *The Book of Life.* W. W. Norton & Co. New York, London. 2001; p 5. Se also his article on Planet of Bacteria, in the *Washington Post Horizons* section 1996(344):H1.

The Plexus Institute conference was Complexity Science, Healthcare and Nursing, was held in Standish, ME from 12 to 14 July 2009.

Paul Ewald. *The Evolution of Infectious Disease.* Oxford University Press, 1994. The information on HIV/AIDS is introduced in this book, but confirmed and elaborated later in personal communications.

Joseph S. Nye Jr. *Soft Power: The Means To Success In World Politics.* Public Affairs Press, 2005.

Much useful information on the down side of antibiotics comes from Dr. J. Douglas Bremner of Emory University School of Medicine and his book: *Before you Take that Pill.* A wide variety of information is available at his web site of the same name: http://www.beforeyoutakethatpill.com.

On the role of friendly GI bacteria see David Mindell. Evolution in the Everyday World. *Scientific American.* Jan. 2009; 300[1]:82-89. Most appropriate is the section on metagenetics.

CHAPTER 7

The Cochran Acute Respiratory Infection Group argument is: Tom Jefferson, Chris Del Mar, Liz Dooley, Eliana Ferroni, Lubna A Al-Ansary, Ghada A Bawazeer, Mieke L van Driel, Ruth Foxlee, Alessandro Rivetti. Physical interventions to interrupt or reduce the spread of respiratory viruses: systematic review. *BMJ* 2009;339:b3675.

Shun-Shin M. Shun-Shin M, Thompson M, Henegen C, et al. Neuraminidase inhibitors for treatment and prophylaxis of influenza in children: systematic review and meta-analysis of randomized controlled trials. *BMJ* 2009;339:b3172.

Those arguing for widespread immunization are, for just one example: Neuzil KM, Zhu Y, Griffin MR, et al. Burden of interpandemic influenza in children younger than five years: a 25 year prospective study. *J Infect Dis* 2002; 185:147-52

On the problem with douching see, for example, Jun Zhang, MB, PhD, A. George Thomas, MD, and Etel Leybovich. Vaginal Douching and Adverse Health Effects: A Meta-Analysis. *Am J Pub Health.* 1997 Jul; 87[7]:1207-11.

CHAPTER 8

The first of the Turku Sugar Studies is: Scheinin A, Makinen KK, Ylitalo K. et al. Turku sugar studies. I. An intermediate report on the effect of sucrose, fructose and xylitol diets on the caries incidence in man. *Acta Odontol Scand.* 1974;32(6):383-412.

An excellent summary of the intervening research is found in: Peldyak J. Makinen KK. Xylitol for caries prevention. *J Dent Hyg.* 2002 Fall;76(4):276-85. The story of xylitol is also told by these authors and myself in a booklet, *Xylitol: A way to better health,* Woodbridge Press, 2004, available through most health food stores.

Tapiainen T, Sormunen R, Kaijalainen T, et al. Ultrastructure of Streptococcus pneumoniae after exposure to xylitol. *J Antimicrob Chemother.* 2004 Jul;54(1):225-8. Epub 2004 Jun 9.

The study showing how the bacteria learn is: Trahan L., Bourgeau G., and Breton R., Emergence of multiple xylitol-resistant (fructose PTS-) mutants from human isolates of mutans streptococci during growth on dietary sugars in the presence of xylitol. *J Dent Res.* 1996 Nov;75(11):1892-1900.

The recent French study looking at dental biofilm is: Badet C, Furiga A, Thébaud N. Effect of xylitol on an in vitro model of oral biofilm. *Oral Health Prev Dent.* 2008;6(4):337-41.

The two studies done in Belize are: Mäkinen KK, Bennett CA, Hujoel PP, Isokangas PJ, Isotupa KP, Pape HR Jr, Mäkinen PL. Xylitol chewing gums and caries rates: a 40-month cohort study. *J Dent Res.* 1995 Dec;74(12):1904-13; and Hujoel PP, Mäkinen KK, Bennett CA, Isotupa KP, Isokangas PJ, Allen P, Mäkinen PL. The optimum time to initiate habitual xylitol gum-chewing for obtaining long-term caries prevention. *J Dent Res.* 1999 Mar; 78(3): 797-803.

Söderling E, Isokangas P, Pienihäkkinen K, Tenovuo J, Alanen P. Influence of maternal xylitol consumption on mother-child transmission of mutans streptococci: 6-year follow-up. *Caries Res.* 2001 May-Jun;35(3):173-7.

Hayes C. The effect of non-cariogenic sweeteners on the prevention of dental caries: a review of the evidence. *J Dent Educ.* 2001 Oct;65(10):1106-9.

CHAPTER 9

Simons D, Brailsford SR, Kidd EA, Beighton D. The effect of medicated chewing gums on oral health in frail older people: a 1-year clinical trial. *J Am Geriatr Soc.* 2002 Aug;50(8):1348-53.

The article that Prof. Hudson refers to is: Hudson VM. Rethinking cystic fibrosis pathology: the critical role of abnormal reduced glutathione (GSH) transport caused by CFTR mutation. *Free Radic Biol Med.* 2001 Jun 15;30(12):1440-61. See also her more recent contribution: Visca A, Bishop CT, Hilton SC, Hudson VM. Improvement in clinical markers in CF patients using a reduced glutathione regimen: an uncontrolled, observational study. *J Cyst Fibros.* 2008 Sep;7(5):433-6. Epub 2008 May 21.

CHAPTER 10

Antonovsky, Aaron. *Unraveling the mystery of health: How people manage stress and stay well.* Jossey-Bass. San Francisco, CA, US: 1987.

Campbell, T. Colin. *The China Study: The Most Comprehensive Study of Nutrition Ever Conducted and the Startling Implications for Diet, Weight Loss and Long-term Health.* Benbella Books. 2006.

For more information on how the idea of adaptation plays out in our current society see our book: Jones, A. H. with Jerry Bozeman. *The Boids and the Bees: Guiding Adaptation to Improve our Health, Health Care, Schools, and Society.* The Institute for the Study of Coherence and Emergence. 2009.

Index

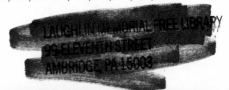

About the Author

Dr. Jones was a clinical assistant professor of family medicine at Texas Tech University Medical School, and practiced at the Hi-Plains Hospital in Hale Center, Texas. He is the inventor and patent-holder of the xylitol-enhanced saline nasal wash/spray sold as Xlear Nasal Wash. Dr.

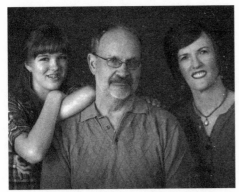

"Lon," as he is referred to by his friends, is a sought-after public speaker on nondrug methods for preventing and reducing upper respiratory conditions. He firmly believes that with xylitol "we have something that can optimize our nasal defenses and help millions of people worldwide."

Dr. Jones with wife Jerry Bozeman and granddaughter Heather

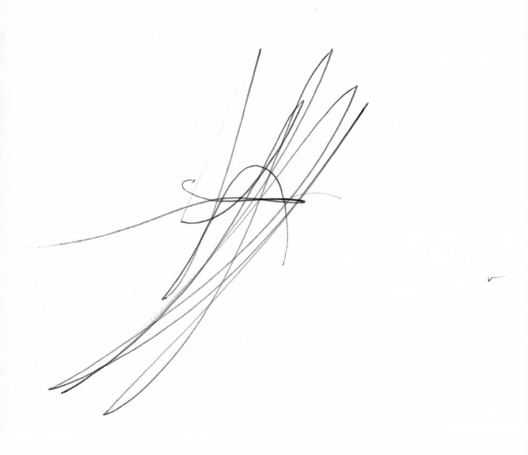

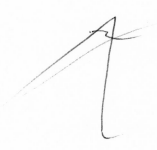